Hard Men Fight Back

Hard Men Fight Back

Kiwi sportsmen who beat the odds to live their dreams

Gregor Paul

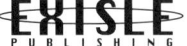

First published 2006

Exisle Publishing Limited,
P.O. Box 60-490, Titirangi, Auckland 1230.
www.exislepublishing.com

Copyright © Gregor Paul 2006
Gregor Paul asserts the moral right to be identified as the author of this work.

All rights reserved. Except for short extracts for the purpose of review, no part of this book may be reproduced, stored in a retrieval system or transmitted in any form or by any means, whether electronic, mechanical, photocopying, recording or otherwise, without prior written permission from the publisher.

National Library of New Zealand Cataloguing-in-Publication Data
Paul, Gregor, 1972-
Hard men fight back : Kiwi sportsmen who beat the odds to live their dream / by Gregor Paul.
ISBN: 0-908988-83-4
1. Athletes-New Zealand. 2. Athletes-Diseases-New Zealand.
3. Athletes-Wounds and injuries-New Zealand. 4. Sport-Psychological aspects. I. Title.
796.0993—dc 22

Text design and production by *BookNZ*
Cover design by Nick Turzynski, redinc., Auckland
Printed in China through Colorcraft Limited, Hong Kong

CONTENTS

| Acknowledgements | 6 |
| Introduction | 7 |

1	Greg Cooper	10
2	Justin Grace	22
3	Kelly Evernden	36
4	Bradley Iles	49
5	Tawera Nikau	64
6	Justin Collins	74
7	Peter Taylor	87
8	Tim Lythe	98
9	Aaron Slight	113
10	Hika Reid	128
11	Eamonn Doyle	140
12	Steve Gurney	153
13	Allan Elsom	165
14	Jeffrey Thumath	174
15	Jared Love	186
16	Michael Utting	198
17	Shane Howarth	212

ACKNOWLEDGEMENTS

It is only when you come to the end of a project such as *Hard Men Fight Back* that you realise how many people have helped along the way. One man who has been there from the start is Exisle's Ian Watt, and I would like to thank him for his support and patience. He shared my vision for this book and was encouraging and positive from the instant he viewed the original proposal.

I want to thank Dr Linda Ashley for giving so generously of her time to share her medical knowledge and display her quite phenomenal eye for detail.

A number of people went above and beyond the call of duty in providing and preparing photographs. Suburban Newspapers were especially helpful and generously provided a number of pictures, including shots taken by the award-winning Fiona Goodall. Others I would like to thank, in no particular order, are Patricia Cooper, John McEwing, Terry Stevenson, Kent Gray, Andrew Cornaga, Jim Hainey, Vinnie Aston, Hannah Johnston, Megan Slight, Graeme Brown, Nigel Marple, Tim Hamilton, Phil Welch, Chris Marriner, Michael Bramley, *The New Zealand Herald* and *Herald on Sunday*.

Lindsay Knight, David Leggat, Dylan Cleaver, Michael Brown and Ron Palenski all dipped into their wealth of sporting knowledge to suggest athletes who would be ideal for this book and Melanie at Celebrity Speakers helped out with some invaluable phone numbers.

To all the coaches, family members and friends who took the time to speak about their loved ones and share what were at times difficult memories, go my sincere and heartfelt thanks. When someone is struck down by a serious illness or injury, the trauma is just as severe and at times worse for close family and friends.

That is why I reserve my final thank you for my wife, Fiona. She was there for me during my own illness and her encouragement, love and support was the foundation stone of this book.

INTRODUCTION

On 17 September 2002 I was diagnosed with testicular cancer. That night I went looking for inspiration to help me through what were going to be the toughest few months of my life.

My search immediately brought me to Lance Armstrong, the American cyclist who at that time had won the Tour de France four times. His victories came after he recovered from testicular cancer that had spread to his lungs and brain. Armstrong had been given only the slimmest chance of living and a few years later he won what is arguably the hardest endurance race in the world. In 2005 Armstrong won a record seventh title and his inspirational story has given hope to thousands of cancer sufferers around the world.

But as I discovered, Armstrong represents only the tip of the iceberg. When I continued my search for high-achieving cancer survivors, I stumbled across legions of athletes who made astonishing sporting comebacks from other serious illnesses, accidents and injuries.

And that is essentially the rationale for this book – I wanted to tell the remarkable stories of New Zealanders who overcame extreme adversity to come back and live out their sporting dreams.

It might seem strange, then, for this book not to feature chapters on either Jonah Lomu or Sir Murray Halberg. Both Halberg and Lomu persevered where others would have given up and both succeeded where others would have failed. They performed at the pinnacle of their respective sports when everyone else said it was impossible. They inspire in the same manner as Armstrong by making us feel that self-belief, hard work and determination will see us through even the most desperate situation.

There is no question that both Lomu and Halberg are iconic, inspirational figures in New Zealand sport. But their intrepid journeys have been well chronicled elsewhere. These pages are devoted to those individuals about whom we know less. Individuals that have displayed the same heroic qualities as Lomu and Halberg without ever enjoying the same recognition. Besides, no doubt once Lomu completes the next phase of his remarkable life, he will commit to print in his own words how he returned to play top-level rugby after a kidney transplant.

Having made the decision to thrust these individuals into the public domain, I can only hope that I have managed to reflect the unassuming nature of all 17. It may come as a surprise to read that not one of the individuals interviewed for this book believed he was worthy of inclusion in a project of this nature. Every athlete I have written about was adamant they had not done anything out of the ordinary, which is probably why so many of these incredible stories have gone largely untold until now.

What also struck me is that all the athletes are linked by the same core attributes. To a man, they all believed they were dealt a fairly awful hand but saw no reason to be bitter. That was crucial, as no one wasted time being angry or raging at his predicament.

Every one of them made a conscious decision to stay positive in the aftermath of his illness or injury. No one was overwhelmed by the length of the road back to the summit of his respective sport. Instead, they all stayed focused on what they wanted to achieve. They all set goals, they all continued to work hard and they all kept believing they would succeed. All these amazing comebacks were driven by a loveable pig-headedness. Everyone who returned to the top of their sport did so because they doggedly refused to pay homage to reality. They had unshakeable visions of an alternative, more positive outcome.

My sincere thanks go to all 17 for giving so generously of their time and for talking so honestly about their lives. It is definitely worth noting that there is another attribute linking them – they are all genuinely good blokes.

Their enthusiasm, warmth and humanity made writing this book so much easier. Special mention must go to Jared Love. When I met him in Hamilton he was living in a garage that belonged to one of his sponsors and he was juggling several jobs to raise the required cash to keep his motorcycling dreams alive. He gave up an afternoon of work to make me feel so very welcome in his humble abode and talk about his life and career with an openness that blew me away.

Not one of the athletes agreed to be interviewed for personal or financial gain or for the vanity value of seeing their name in print. They gave of their time because they liked the idea that by doing so they could inspire others less fortunate than themselves.

They needn't worry on that front. Their courage, determination and tenacity make compelling reading. I can only hope that my words do their endeavours justice. What I am sure of is that these incredible people fill us all with hope that should we find ourselves in a similar hole, we too can climb out of it stronger and more rounded for the experience.

I was moved listening to the testimony of every athlete. I will resist the temptation to make special mention of any one person, as I think it is obvious from the writing that follows the high regard in which I hold them all.

Instead, I would like to make reference to three people. I found listening to Greg Cooper recount how he was taken home to die as a teenager particularly emotional. Given virtually no hope of surviving, he was an All Black by the age of 21.

Eamonn Doyle's conversion from listless teenager into a national indoor rowing champion was almost too incredible to believe. The catalyst for this extraordinary conversion was a horrific motorcycle crash that put him in a coma for four weeks and a rehabilitation centre for six months. At the time of going to print Eamonn was desperately hoping to get some indication as to whether he could be in the frame to serve as a crew member on Team New Zealand's 2007 America's Cup bid.

Perhaps, though, the individual who could provide the most inspirational comeback of all is track athlete Jeffrey Thumath. This young man has suffered more than anyone should. Diagnosed with testicular cancer at 17, Jeffrey has been in and out of hospital for the last three years, enduring chemotherapy and several serious bouts of surgery. In January 2006 he finally got the all-clear to make a full return to athletics. No one could be more deserving of a lift in fortune and it would take the coldest heart not to melt should Jeffrey fulfil his dream of competing at the 2010 Commonwealth Games.

Jeffrey, like the other 16 athletes in this book, is a reluctant hero. But heroes are most definitely what they all are.

Gregor Paul
March 2006

1

GREG COOPER

All Black 1986–1992

Greg Cooper made a pathetic figure as he tottered towards the hayshed on the family farm. His skeletal frame was almost buckling from the sheer effort of simply keeping itself upright. The emaciated face and hollow, black eyes were obvious signs the chemotherapy and radiotherapy had taken their toll.

His father watched, his heart tearing at the seams. Cooper was just 16 years old, horribly sick and not a great bet to make it to his 17th birthday.

But while the body was weak, the mind was strong. Driving Cooper's stick-thin legs into that makeshift weights room in the hayshed was the total conviction that one day he would be an All Black. However ridiculous, however unlikely, Cooper could not be swayed from his belief that at some stage in his life he would stand proud in black. He had been given a 10 per cent chance of living and he was thinking about winning test caps.

He never once thought about dying. He wanted to live too much and the idea that something was trying to take that away stoked the fires within.

That rage helped him. It helped him get through the challenge of hoisting the bar 10 times. Achieving every goal was vital if he was to get his weight back before the next bout of chemotherapy. At the end of each cycle he'd come home and weigh himself. It was always 64 kg. His normal weight was 76 kg. That was the challenge, then. To get up to 76 kg before the next infusion of toxins.

Each time he came into the hayshed, he would stand under the bar and close his eyes. Then he would lose himself in his thoughts – the same dream every time. He'd be standing with his All Black team-mates, singing the national anthem, feeling the nervous excitement that would be inevitable on his test debut. As the words to *God Defend New Zealand* swirled round the stadium, he'd begin his session, tears streaming down his cheeks. For someone so sick and so young, he played a lot of test football.

Since being diagnosed with Ewing's Sarcoma (bone cancer) in February 1981, Cooper's life had been simplified so he could focus on just two things. The first was survival. The second was playing test football. It was as if the two goals had become one. They were no longer mutually exclusive. Survival, he was sure, would lead to an All Black call-up. Cooper didn't care that his life had become locked into a cycle that saw him traipse from hospital to home, from home to hospital. He had been taken out of school, such was the toll of his treatment. And yet, none of this could persuade him that he may have been just a touch ambitious with his goal-setting.

He knew his destiny the instant he learned of his prognosis – a diagnosis had been made after he complained of suffering from an excruciatingly sore shoulder on a family holiday to Australia. Once back in New Zealand, his mother took him to hospital. He knew he was in a lot of pain. He knew there was a problem of some magnitude. He was told death was lurking six months down the track. When the surgeons informed his parents, Pat and Patricia, that a tumour had been found on the upper right rib, an inoperable spot, they were asked whether they wanted to be the ones to tell their son his chances of survival were not good. Pretty bad in fact. It was a horrible moment, probably the hardest thing any parent could ever do.

'Greg was pretty upset, as you would expect,' remembers Patricia. 'He cried for a little bit and then all of a sudden he just said he wasn't going to die and he was going to be an All Black.

'Greg had always been very strong. Even as a small child he had been very strong and he just never accepted that he wasn't going to be all right. Things were so bad they weren't even going to give him chemotherapy or radiotherapy, but in the end I guess they just decided they would anyway.'

Cooper's conviction he would become an All Black was not random. In the season preceding his diagnosis, as a strapping 15-year-old, he was good enough to play for the First XV at St John's College, Hastings, and the dream of making it to the test arena had already taken seed. When the tumour was found, that dream was brought out of the dark recesses at the back of Cooper's mind and placed firmly in the forefront. It was the way he coped with the disease. The brain was immediately installed as the general in the battle against cancer. Its strategy was built on positive thinking: eradicate the negative and send only positive vibes to the blood cells on the front line.

To this day Cooper's not too sure how his mind became so resolute. 'I don't know if I was naive or very fortunate, but there was never one time in all of that when I thought I wasn't going to come through, even though the outlook was bleak. The doctors never said that to me, they only said it to my parents. It was probably a good thing because my outlook was only positive. I believe in the power of the mind. If my mind was strong and being boosted by my body being strong, then I could fight the illness. It wasn't if I was going to get well, it was always when, even during the deepest, darkest moments.'

And there were plenty of dark moments. Of course there were. Cancer is at its most evil when it strikes in children. It's usually the sneakiest devil, too, giving little warning of its presence. The only indications Cooper had that things weren't all as they should be came in Australia and a few weeks earlier in the gym when he found it hard to grip the weights bar. The tumour was pressing on a nerve to his arm. A weak wrist doesn't prepare you for the news that you have cancer. Shock is the obvious and indeed only reaction. And it's a shock that can take some time to absorb. Yet,

Greg Cooper

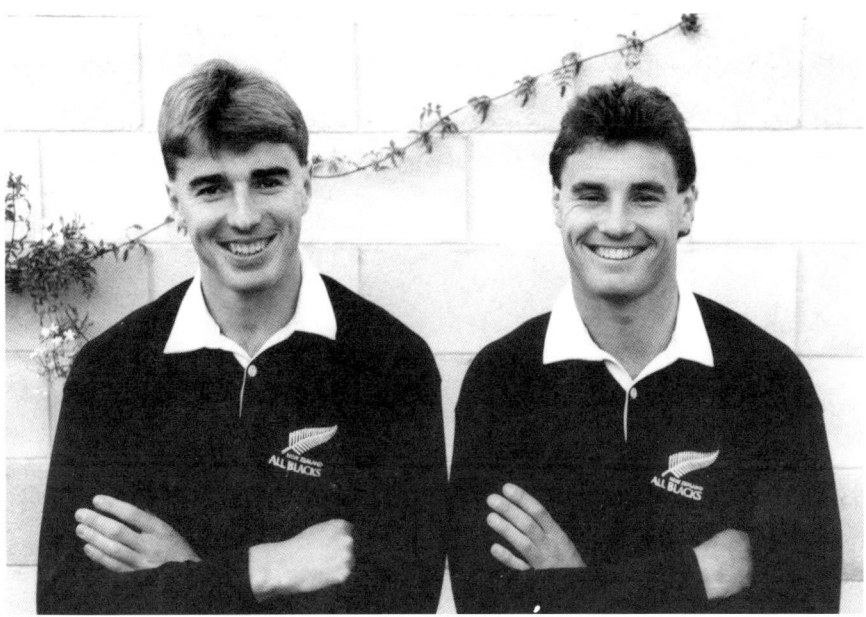

Greg Cooper and his brother Matthew pose in their All Black jerseys in 1992. *Patricia Cooper*

strangely, it's not the disease that knocks the sufferer for six. Cancer, in many ways, is a pussy-cat compared with chemotherapy. The drugs take no prisoners. The toxins swish through the veins wiping out anything that gets in their path. Cooper didn't react well to his treatment. The vomiting was constant. The tiredness could never be slept away.

'Unfortunately, the mass of tissue was on the first rib, in an area where surgical removal was impossible. The word to my parents was to take him home and in six to eight months you are going to have a very sick boy on your hands. I ended up having six weeks of radiotherapy and two years of chemotherapy.

'I used to say to myself if what is going into my body is designed to kill the cancer, as bad as I feel, the cancer must be feeling worse. As long as I could handle it, I wanted as much as I could. It was an internal battle. I started feeling sick and I started saying, "I know you are inside me. I'm harder than you are, I'll last longer than you."'

To his family and friends, Cooper's optimism was admirable, a testament to his courage. But realism figured in their thinking. They knew the odds of survival. They could see the physical toll. Prior to being diagnosed, Cooper was running seven kilometres back from school. Every day he got a little faster, recording his best time the day before the hammer blow was dealt. After a couple of months of chemotherapy, once-powerful arms hung like withered twigs. Legs that were bounding over acres of farmland only weeks earlier looked like they could snap in a stiff wind. It seemed a hopeless task diverting death from its inevitable path.

Cooper just couldn't accept that, though. His faith was not going to be shaken. Patricia remembers coming to visit him in Palmerston North while he was having chemotherapy. 'I remember the sister taking me into the ward and then finding an empty bed and asking people if they had seen Greg Cooper anywhere. Someone said he had gone out running. She was pretty furious and started saying how Greg shouldn't even be walking, let alone running.

'But that was Greg. He had this theory that if he could get oxygen round his body it would help fight the cancer. I don't know if there was any scientific fact to support that but he believed it and the doctors were quite happy for him to run as they thought it was best for Greg to deal with things in his own way.

'I can also remember phoning his sister who he was staying with in Palmerston North while having treatment. She would tell me she was fitter than she had ever been. When I asked why she told me that Greg had been out running almost every day. She said she couldn't let him go out there on his own, so she went with him.

'It was strange in a way because I knew how sick Greg was. We could see how ravaged he was by the treatment. His legs and face were so terribly thin and he was so weak. But I never really felt he was going to die. I think Greg was just so positive, so strong and always telling us how he was going to be an All Black that we couldn't equate death with our boy.'

By keeping himself physically active, it meant that all the time in his head, Cooper was winning. He was going to survive. He wasn't going to give an inch. He wasn't going to lose control. The strength of his mind would determine the strength of his body. And what kept his mind in control was his conviction he was going to become an All Black.

'I had a goal to get my weight to where it was before I was sick. I was basically staying in a holding pattern. But if I didn't do it, I would lose too much weight and not be able to fight the illness. Although I might have started my chemotherapy at 76 kg and come out at 64 kg, by the time I was ready for more treatment I was back at 76 kg through running and weight training. But I always knew that in two days' time, bang, I was going to go down to 64 kg. I viewed that as a far better option than going back in at 57 kg.

'I remember one day Dad saw me looking skeletal and I remember him saying "I wish that was me". But I didn't want him to be in that situation. I could handle it and I kept thinking "Thank God it's me and not him".

'I see goals as a pathway. I look at dreams as being the emotive side of a goal. And I had a vision. When I was at home and had spent a couple of days feeling really rough from the effects of chemotherapy, I would put the weights bar on my shoulders and start squatting. As I was working, I would see myself in that black jersey and I could see myself singing the national anthem and that would get me to the 10th repetition.'

After the first few months of treatment, he was allowed to go back to school. It helped him establish normality. It gave the illusion he was just another teenager, getting on with his life. The bald head was a bit of a giveaway that he wasn't normal. It said that he wasn't like the other kids, but no one was cruel. That was important. Acceptance allowed him to believe he could carry on where he left off before his diagnosis. There wasn't anyone reminding him of his plight. Probably the last thing he needed was to have his battle thrust in his face either by well-wishers or those with a more twisted motive.

Once back at school and surrounded by his peer group, the desire to be out playing rugby became overwhelming. His medical team were understandably reluctant to sanction the move. He was, after all, still receiving serious dosages of chemotherapy. He needed his energy to cope with that and fight the disease, not chase a ball round a muddy paddock.

But Cooper's passion burned so brightly inside, it could easily be seen. As his weight began to stabilise between chemotherapy cycles, he was given permission to switch to monthly sessions, enabling him to play some football. His doctors took the view that it would have done more harm to his mental wellbeing if they had prevented him from playing. They had also come to realise that trying to stop him would have been futile. To have said no would only have made Cooper more determined. And anyway, what harm could it do?

His return to rugby was far from glorious. He was so keen to make an impact that he had only managed 10 minutes in his comeback game when he split his eye open trying to knock somebody into next week. It required stitching and therefore another trip to the hospital, a journey whose familiarity had most definitely bred contempt. Given what he had been through, a facial cut was hardly going to knock the wind out of his sails. Worse followed, however. In his next game he again tried to flatten everything that came near him. His shoulder was the next casualty. It required a reconstruction. There was more frustration, more setbacks, but still he believed. Still he saw his name on that All Black team sheet.

The first sign that his luck was turning, that maybe his dream really could be fulfilled, came in his penultimate year at school when he was selected to play for New Zealand Schools. It was an incredible achievement, especially as he was still receiving treatment at the time. He had been diagnosed almost two years earlier and still the poison was being pumped into his system.

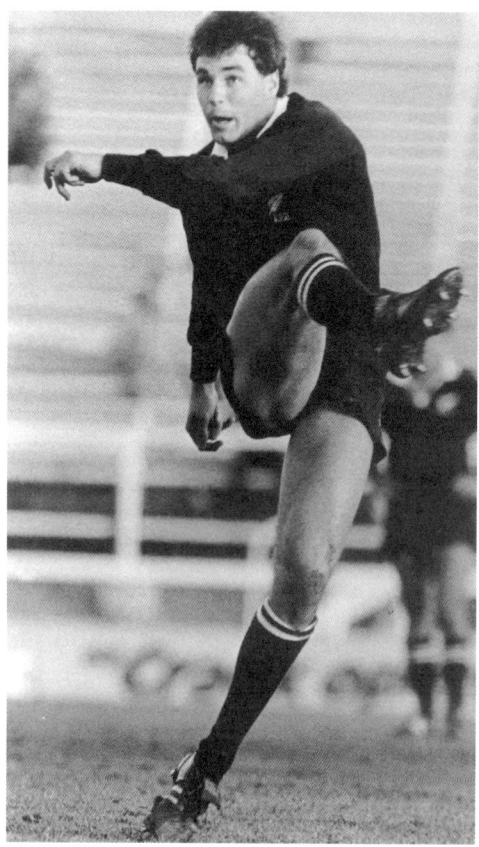

Greg Cooper kicks for goal in his All Black debut against France. *New Zealand Herald*

There needed to be a cut-off point. A time when the doctors simply said enough is enough. His young, developing body was at breaking point. Patricia, though, didn't want the treatment to stop.

'The instant the needle came out of Greg's arm in the hospital he would ask me to take him home. I can remember the family all going to bed and Greg and I going downstairs and he would lie on the couch. I would have a bucket to hold for him and he would be so sick. I would count for three minutes and there would be nothing left to come out of him. Just bile and he would still be retching. This would go on all night.

'It was really very hard for Greg but I didn't want them to stop giving him the treatment. I thought if they stopped the treatment that would be it. But the doctors felt Greg had had enough. That his body needed a break.'

Once the treatment had been stopped, the Cooper family and his doctors were all desperately hoping for the miracle. Desperately hoping they would find some evidence that the body was responding. They got it when an X-ray showed the bone in his rib had grown back and hardened up.

When Cooper had first been diagnosed the bone was a mushy pulp. The X-ray wasn't reason to declare victory, but it was certainly a positive sign that Cooper's body was beginning to rebuild itself. But cancer is a dogged opponent. It can often appear as if it has given up, only to strike back. That's why sufferers can never relax. Cooper, at least, could stop his treatment. Think beyond getting through each cycle. Never, though, did his thoughts stray beyond an All Black jersey.

'It was probably an obsession, but I think it was an obsession that was easy to understand. To make the All Blacks was like saying to everyone around me and anyone that cared about me that I had beaten cancer. Decisions were made in the interests of trying to become an All Black.

'I wanted to get somewhere in a hurry and I was selected in the Hawke's Bay squad after I left school and played the first game. But the selectors told me after that game that no matter how well I played, I was too young. As a coach now I can understand where they were coming from, but I was not your normal 18-year-old. I had just been through two or three very tough years and I wanted to be an All Black the next day. And being told no matter how well I played was not going to make any difference … I don't think they could quite comprehend where I was coming from. My world was a different world. Halfway through the season the chance came up to go to Otago and achieve what I wanted to achieve. Cancer does give you more resolve to achieve what you have always wanted to achieve.'

That chance came up because soon-to-be All Black coach John Hart had seen Cooper play for New Zealand Schools. He was impressed enough to then select Cooper for his New Zealand Barbarians side. The Barbarians played Otago and Cooper had a convincing game at fullback. There were whispers that the interest of the Otago coaching staff had been piqued, so after Hawke's Bay had made their position clear, Cooper enrolled at Otago University.

The studying, however, was not his main reason for shifting south. He was really going down to try and make it into Otago's NPC team. If he did, it would put him in front of the national selectors every week. Perhaps unsurprisingly, the studying soon fell by the wayside. It was getting in the way of his obsession. The decks had to be clear. The mind focused on that one goal. It helped. His form for Otago was consistently good. He was earning recognition. But by 1986 he was so homesick he shifted up to Auckland. He needed to be nearer his family. They had been his foundation throughout his battle with cancer. The bond linking the Coopers was strong. Strong enough for Cooper to realise he needed to have that support network nearby if he was going to succeed in his mission.

The shift to Auckland came with another massive attraction. The Aucks, at that time, could lay claim to being one of the greatest provincial sides in New Zealand's history. They were loaded with big name All Blacks such as Sean Fitzpatrick, Gary and Alan Whetton, John Kirwan, Steve McDowell and Michael Jones. If Cooper could break into the starting fifteen he would be knocking on the door of test selection. That was how it was – if you were good enough to play for Auckland at that time, then you really weren't far off being ready to play for the All Blacks. As the season progressed, Cooper was holding down a starting place and looking every inch a test candidate for the number 15 jersey.

It helped that 1986 loomed as a year of opportunity. The rebel tour of South Africa had thrust New Zealand rugby into turmoil. A number of top players, first choice All Blacks, had ignored a New Zealand Rugby Union edict by travelling to South Africa to play an unofficial test series. Those who travelled to the Republic were banned from playing for the All Blacks. As a consequence, a number of places in the national team were up for grabs.

And so it was, against all the odds, five years after he first dragged his ailing body into the makeshift weights room on the family farm, Cooper got the call so many had never dared believe would come. All those nights he had spent retching over a bucket, all the suffering and mental anguish. It hadn't been in vain. He had been selected to play for the All Blacks against France at Lancaster Park, Christchurch on 28 June. His knees wobbled a bit when he heard the news, the tears welled up, but he stayed staunch. Permission for his bottom lip to quiver was firmly denied.

'I was at Wellington Airport when a reporter rang me. I think it was Don Cameron. The first thing I wanted to do was phone Mum and Dad. I was trying not to be too emotional. It was almost like me paying them back. I thought it must be a good feeling for them to see me make the All Blacks. It was my way of saying thanks for all that help they had given me.

'When I ran out against France in 1986 it almost felt strange. It felt as though I had been there before because the dream was so vivid. It was an emotional day. I was on a complete high. I hardly did anything wrong. It was almost as if I knew the game was going to go my way. I hit one of the best dropkicks I have ever hit to go 3-0 up. Not that I ever thought it at the time, but maybe I did say to myself "now it's over".'

For his family, who were all at Lancaster Park, it was almost impossible to believe the teenager who had been at death's door, almost rung the bell in fact, had now been selected to represent the country's most elite group of athletes. Not so long ago he had been a 64 kg bag of bones.

'I can remember it was surreal,' says Patricia. 'Of course we were all so proud of Greg and amazed that he had done it but I just couldn't take it in. I couldn't take in that this was the same boy who had been so sick.

This was the same boy who we had been told to take home to die. People probably don't realise that Greg has no muscle in his right shoulder. When he wears a suit it has padding, but when he takes it off there is only a tiny bit of muscle that the surgeons left him. It was an incredible story. A wonderful story.'

That game in Christchurch brought Cooper closure. It closed the book on what had been an extraordinary fight. A fight he had won, enabling him to claim the ultimate prize – his life. He'd been given a 10 per cent chance of surviving. His dream of becoming an All Black had always appeared slightly ridiculous. As he thundered all over Lancaster Park five years later, it seemed utterly ridiculous that as a 15-year-old, as he had been when he was initially diagnosed, he had been so close to death.

He earned six more caps before he eventually hung his boots up in 1996. Maybe it could have been more. But that was never what Cooper's career was about. It was about proving to himself and those who knew him that adversity could not stop him. That he could achieve his ultimate goals in life no matter how unlikely others rated his chances.

In 2005 he was again defying the odds, this time as coach of the Highlanders Super 12 side. The so-called experts reckoned the Highlanders were a certainty for the wooden spoon. Not for the first time in his life, Cooper had other ideas. He never doubted his ability as a coach and never believed what others were saying.

He stayed true to his own beliefs, his own values, and instilled a work ethic and character into his team that was the mirror image of himself. His reward was to take his side to the brink of the play-offs and ram large helpings of humble pie down the throats of those who had written them off.

His character has been shaped by his experience in defeating cancer. The experience will always be with him. Not dominating his thoughts, but always helping shape them, always providing that little extra belief that he can succeed in every aspect of his life. If there is a downside, he feels that perhaps he focused too hard on becoming an All Black. He had his eye on one day and never thought much beyond it.

'I'm not saying I would ever have become a great All Black. From my cancer days I have one lung with reduced capacity because of the radiotherapy. The doctors told my parents I would never run again. I also have quite severe damage round one shoulder. There were some physical limitations. It would have been hard for me to make it into the top echelon of players. But I set myself a goal to reach the finish line, not go past it.

'I don't have any regrets. I am very fortunate to have had even one test match. If I had my time again, maybe, just maybe, I would have seen past that first match. But again if somebody said to me that is the only test you will ever play, I would have been a very happy man. It wasn't about being a great All Black. It was about completing a goal I had set myself.'

He says he wasn't a legendary All Black. Others may well disagree.

Greg Cooper played seven tests at fullback for the All Blacks between 1986 and 1992, scoring 63 points. His provincial career stretched across 12 years, in which time he represented Hawke's Bay, Auckland and Otago. He went on to amass a record 1520 points for Otago. At the tail end of his playing career he was drafted into the Auckland Blues Super 12 team and played three professional games in the 1996 season. He moved into coaching in 2001, holding positions first with Otago then the Highlanders, where he remains today. In 2006 he was also appointed coach of the New Zealand Under-21 team. He lives in Dunedin with wife Sam and children Hannah, Ben and Alexandra.

2

JUSTIN GRACE

New Zealand Commonwealth Games Sprint Cycling Team 2002 and 2006

When Justin Grace clambered off his bike in Bogota, he knew he could no longer delay the inevitable. The pain was searing. The stomach cramps were so severe that just standing up was an ordeal. The bleeding was heavy and it took just a glance at the ghostly complexion to know he was badly anaemic.

Since the age of 17 he'd known this day would come. The day when his illness would have to be granted the attention it so desperately craved.

For almost eight years he had kept the surgeon's knife at bay. He hadn't so much been in denial as in defiance, determined to succeed in professional sprint cycling even though the odds were stacked against him.

Living with ulcerative colitis was never easy. But Grace had always managed to keep it at arm's length. His training regime was brutal, capable of breaking any athlete who had just a hint of doubt about their dedication. To be able to clock less than 11 seconds over 200 m on the track, Grace had to punish every muscle and every organ. That made him no different to any other elite cyclist. It is a cruel and demanding sport that doesn't reward the half-hearted or those who think they can take a short cut to the top.

What made him different was that he was competing with an illness that really gave him no right to be performing at that level. Since his diagnosis at the end of 1987 he couldn't go for more than 45 minutes without needing the toilet. There would be bad days where his every waking moment would be spent wishing he was in bed. There he would be able to ride out the stomach cramps that swept across him like crashing waves. There he could just shut his eyes and take his mind on a journey away from the grim reality. The truth was that a mixed genetic hand had blessed him with the talent to operate at the elite level of world cycling, yet it had also inflicted him with a disease that would prevent him from ever fulfilling his potential. As he advanced into his early twenties, the training and competition were beginning to take their toll. His body was struggling to handle the workload and as much as he didn't want it to be true, a voice inside was screaming, begging him to give up his dream and accept that his illness had destined him for a role as an average Joe.

There had been more than a few occasions when he had nearly obeyed the voice. Since the age of 11 he had been driven by his desire to be a cycling great. As a schoolboy in Pukekohe he won national titles and planted himself on the radar of the sport's senior selectors.

But as a hugely promising 16-year-old, just a few weeks before the national road championships, he started to feel jaded. It wasn't bad enough to worry about, but he was aware everything was not as it should have been. He didn't dwell on it, but when it came to race day, he couldn't quite squeeze out everything in his tank and finished, for him, a disappointing fifth. It was hugely frustrating – knowing he could have done better but not being able to capitalise on all the hard work he had invested.

Normality didn't kick in after the road champs. His health deteriorated almost as fast as he propelled his bike and he was no longer able to keep the issue a nagging doubt. It was now very much in his face.

As Grace recalls: 'The next year, 1987, I was doing an apprenticeship. For the first three months I was very, very sick. I knew something was really wrong. I had bad stomach cramps. I had to go to the toilet every 45 minutes. I was tired all the time and I felt like I needed to be in bed 24 hours a day. But I was trying to make a start in the world. I wasn't racing well. It took until the end of the year until I got a diagnosis. Because of my age they weren't looking for ulcerative colitis.'

His diagnosis gave him relief of sorts. While it was hardly good news to find out he was suffering from a debilitating disease that would have a detrimental impact on his ability to succeed in his chosen sport, it was at least an answer as to why he had been feeling so awful. With understanding of his problem he could manage it. He could fight it and determine his boundaries.

It was never that simple, though. He was trying to forge a living as a professional cyclist. He was based in Canada and spending months at a time in various training camps, living out of a suitcase and taking his body to breaking point almost every day. It's a cut-throat world where no one can afford to be off their game even by a fraction of a second. With the margin between success and failure so thin, every possible means of extracting a competitive advantage has to be explored, especially if the difference between winning and losing is linked to financial security.

Grace was operating in such a demanding environment, yet he had major problems dealing with some very basic issues. There were problems with fluid intake, replacement of electrolytes and vitamin deficiencies. In 1990 he started taking drugs to ease the symptoms. They made it more tolerable, made him feel better about himself. There were associated problems with his medication, however. They had unpleasant side-effects and he also needed dispensation from the sport's administrators to use them. Because of this he tried to take them as little as possible. And as a consequence of not taking his medication, he says, 'I had three really crap years. A lot of people said as soon as I was diagnosed that I should have stopped racing right there and then. I didn't think about it then. But there was a period in 1994 when I was ready to give it all up. I was finishing outside the top five regularly and I knew I was better than that. I found that really frustrating.

'It all came to a head after I had been in Cuba for a couple of months. We were hammered while we were over there and everyone got sick. I didn't handle it too well. When I came home I was so sick and I thought

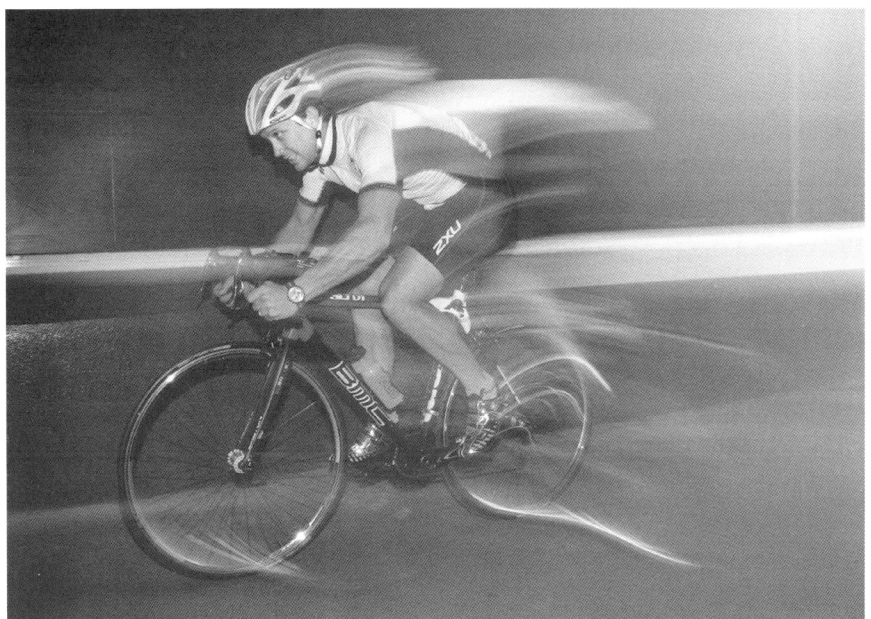

Justin Grace poses outside his Newmarket bike shop in February 2006 as he prepares for the Commonwealth Games in Melbourne. *Chris Skelton, Herald on Sunday*

I was stupid doing this. I thought I shouldn't be doing it to myself any more. I was going to pack it in and ride motorbikes so I didn't have to pedal. I even got as far as testing bikes to see which one I liked and what class I was going to ride in.

'But I was due to cycle in the Canadian national championships later that year. My dad had booked to come over and he was pretty disappointed that he wasn't going to see me race. I started to feel better and decided to go for fun. Once I got there, for the first time in my career I rode 11 seconds. It persuaded me to carry on and I rode the nationals and finished third. I got some motivation to go home and look after myself after that. To train properly and refocus my goals.'

Making the 1996 Olympics in Atlanta became the number one priority. Once again, though, Grace's physical condition was at odds with his ambition. As much as he wanted to make it to the States, his surgeon wasn't so sure. He felt the time had come to remove Grace's large intestine, an operation many sufferers of ulcerative colitis have to undergo at some point. The disease ulcerates the lining of the intestine and causes extensive bleeding and dramatically increases the risk of bowel cancer, particularly if it goes untreated over a long period.

Grace needed a stay of execution to preserve his Olympic dream. He got it at the 1995 Pan American Games in Argentina. His condition stabilised enough for him to finish fifth in the sprints.

It was an impossibly good performance in Argentina. So much at odds with his deteriorating health that maybe someone should invent the Grace Formula to explain other cases where athletic performance proves to be inversely proportional to health.

His Olympic dream was real. Whatever his blood tests said, the stadium clocks were disagreeing. It would have been too cruel to kill his dream, so once again the surgeon backed off.

The World Championships in Bogota, Colombia at the end of 1995 would be Grace's judgement day. Colombia was his chance to qualify for the Olympics. He arrived in South America in awful physical condition but a superb state of mind.

He left in even worse physical condition and his spirit was crushed, too, when he rode like a demon only to miss out on Atlanta by .0003 of a second. It really wasn't any kind of consolation to be able to say he would have been the next cab off the rank if an Olympic vacancy became available.

But by the time he was high above the Bogota smog, his only thought was to get to Auckland and throw himself into the arms of his medical team.

'I was very sick at that stage. I flew home through Canada and I rang my dad to tell the surgeon I wasn't going to the Olympics. I flew home not knowing what was going to happen. Within a couple of weeks I was in hospital in Auckland and it was a bit of a blur. I didn't think it was going to be such a big thing.

'I had been hardcore racing and I left a bunch of stuff over at my North American base and I still haven't been back to get it. I thought I would need all that stuff soon. The surgery was so much more difficult to deal with than I thought. They took my whole large intestine out and a small piece of the small intestine. I had to have a colostomy bag for three months.'

Well, it would have been for three months if everything had gone to plan. It didn't. About five weeks after the initial surgery, Grace was not recovering as he should. He was still tired, still weak and struggling.

He was called back into Mercy Hospital. They wanted to observe him. He was put on a drip, getting weaker by the minute. After a few days they decided there was no option but to open him up again. The problem was the scar tissue. It wasn't healing to the doctors' satisfaction. It was no one's fault. Just bad luck. It was a big call to open him up again. Even prime athletes can't breeze through two major bouts of surgery in the space of five weeks. There wasn't a lot of choice, though. Once he came round, it was a case of wait and see. Cross fingers and hope the problems had been fixed. Hope that Grace would begin his journey back to normality.

That hope was proving forlorn. By Christmas Eve, any gamblers would have had their money on the Grim Reaper. If Grace had been asked to make a call back then, probably he too would have slipped a few bob on him meeting his maker.

Estimating how many hours you are away from death is hardly an exact science, or a skill in which one would like to become adept, but Grace feels he could not have lasted another 12 hours. His aunt, who had visited him earlier in the day, felt the same way. She had called Grace's father after her visit, to advise him to gather the family. He was 24, far too young to be the subject of a bedside vigil.

'I knew that if I didn't start getting better in the next 12 hours I was not going to survive. It was amazing. Just like the movies where people say gather the family around. I really understood what those weak people feel. I really thought I was going to die. I had tubes up my nose, down my throat. There were wires everywhere. I could hardly move. All night there was this green goo coming out of me for hours and hours.

'I hadn't eaten anything for days. It was really nasty. It is very difficult to explain what it feels like. You can say the words but they don't really mean anything. It's a bit like when you are holding on to monkey bars. There comes a time when you know you can start counting down from 10 because you are not going to be able to hold on any longer. That's pretty much where I was. I knew I couldn't do it for another 12 hours.'

He owes his survival to that same invisible force that had been propelling him round cycle tracks faster than he had any right to travel. Call it determination. Call it passion. Call it what you like – there is something programmed into the core of Grace that makes him one of life's fighters.

Others would have slipped into unconsciousness and quietly moved on to the next world. Not Grace. He'd been fighting for the last seven years. Every day had been a massive struggle. Christmas Eve 1995 was not so different; just a bit tougher than the norm, a day which required Grace to dig a little deeper into his well of defiance. By morning, the nurse who sat by his bed all night reported a distinct improvement in Grace's condition when the doctors came through on their morning rounds.

It was that fighting instinct which Grace's father, Murray, knew would save his son. Ever since Justin had first jumped on a bike as an 11-year-old, he'd seen the determination. It was as much a source of concern as it was pride. He'd always harboured a secret wish Grace would just give it all up. Stop pushing himself so hard and give his body the break it needed. He'd never said it, though. He didn't want to be discouraging. He didn't want to do anything to stop his son chasing his goal. He also knew that if he had ever said anything, his advice would have been immediately ignored. Grace was driven and his father knew it.

'I always felt Justin would get better,' is Grace senior's matter-of-fact recollection. 'I remember his auntie phoning me after she visited and she said he'd thrown the towel in, that he had given up. But I never thought that. Justin was always pushing himself.

'It was a bit of a shock, though. When he came out of the first surgery, the surgeon said they'd got him just in time. He wouldn't have wanted to put the operation off any longer.'

The surgeon, Mischel Neill, would later tell Grace how he was amazed that he was even managing to function as a normal person, let alone holding down a world ranking of 35.

Grace had survived the second round of surgery. Albeit only just, but his dream of competing in a major cycling championship had been shattered. His old life was dead. He felt a little foolish having been so naive as to think he would be back on his bike within 12 months. He most certainly was not going to be picking up where he left off. His world ranking of 35 when he staggered out of Bogota was as good as it was ever going to get.

And if he didn't know it when he walked out of Mercy Hospital, he knew it 18 months later when he hopped back into the saddle.

'It was very hard for my body to get used to the new way of working. I was in really peak physical condition and lost 11 kilos through that surgery. I was fit and strong and knew how to make myself hurt. I thought within a year I would be back. In 1996 I watched everything in the Olympics apart from the cycling. I couldn't bear to watch it.

'Six months on I was still exhausted walking up the driveway. A year down the track I was starting to live a reasonably normal life but something still didn't quite feel right. About 18 months down the track I thought I would start to ride. But after two or three days I would start to get a bit sick. My body just couldn't handle it.

'It took me about two years to get over the surgery and maybe realise that I was never going to race again. I had spent my whole life since I was 11 racing. I didn't ride for a total of six years. I just enjoyed being a normal person and having money and being able to buy things. I kind of enjoyed doing that – not having cycling in my life – after struggling all those years. I met my wife and we got married. Life was good.'

And just like that, Grace buried his desire to conquer the cycling world. The voice that had been nagging away for all those years had finally won. Strangely, it wasn't so bad. He didn't miss the training. The sheer brutality of building his body up and smashing it down didn't hold the same appeal. There was, as Grace was discovering, much more to life than pedalling his body beyond its limits.

His health was pretty good. There were good days and bad days, but things seemed more manageable now. So good, that in 2000 he felt comfortable buckling to peer pressure from his work colleagues and joining them in a few triathlons. Not surprisingly, he did the cycle legs.

His wife, Erika, was a regular in the gym, so Grace joined her. He was getting fit. Not for any purpose, just for the joy of it. And as he began to enjoy it more, every now and again his thoughts would drift, just slightly, but they would drift back to the old days. Were they really gone? Would he really have to go to his grave wondering what might have been? Of course he would. There is a world of difference between having fun at local triathlons and whizzing round velodromes at the same speed as the best cyclists in the world.

Whenever the thoughts started to drift, they were reined in before they were able to roam free. They were always cut off at the pass, as it were, so they couldn't manifest into anything more serious.

Imperceptibly, though, he began to increase his efforts in the gym. Nothing major, just a few extra minutes here and there. A bit more effort in the final stages of every session.

He did so with fear as his companion. It lived with him every turn of the pedals. He was terrified that his body, by now a semi-reliable machine, would throw a wobbly when asked to step out of its comfort zone. He kept waiting for the stomach cramps to kick in. He kept waiting for that overwhelming tiredness to grab him at work. He kept waiting, but nothing happened. By September 2001 his thoughts were drifting on a daily basis, buoyed by his ever-improving fitness and health. He decided that maybe it was better to die trying than to die wondering. He would know more about his ability, both physical and mental, if he put himself through an exhaustive 10-week training programme.

'I was really enjoying it so I decided I might start trying a little harder. I was just pushing myself a little bit more. I was expecting the wheels to fall off but they didn't. So I would try a little bit harder. We got to September 2001 and I decided I was going to train for eight to 10 weeks really hard and see what happened. I was terrified after being sick for so many years. I didn't want to fail again. I'm not the sort of person who likes failing.

'For the first two years after my surgery, I had lived my life as a normal person. I was thinking I was going to be an average Joe. But after riding with Erika and doing a few triathlons I was feeling pretty good. I simulated a training camp we had done before the Commonwealth Games. I was taking half days at work and training in the morning and at night. I was feeling good and putting on weight.'

His self-imposed training camp finished just as the track season was beginning in early 2002. He felt as good, if not better, than at any point in his pre-surgery career. Plenty of athletes, though, have felt invincible after tough training camps only to come horribly unstuck in competition. So it was with no expectations that Grace headed down to Wanganui for the International Night of the Stars meeting in January 2002.

How could it be any other way? He hadn't raced competitively for almost seven years. He was going to be riding on his old bike. It was almost as much a relic as Grace. Man and machine had both seen the sport advance to new levels while they contemplated their respective new lives – one coming to terms with life as a mere mortal, the other put out to pasture in the garage. Only a fool would be riding with hope.

In Wanganui Grace rode a personal-best time at sea level of 10.71 seconds in the sprint. His whole career had been about defying the odds. This, though, well, this was taking the piss. And from the instant Grace's front wheel crossed the line, his whole life became about one thing.

'At that stage I decided to make the Commonwealth Games in Manchester my number one goal. I told my wife and she told me not to be ridiculous. But I knew things were going really well and it went from there. I told my gastro specialist and he said not to overdo it. My blood tests were all looking good.

'I know enough other athletes to know they all feel the same about their sport. There is something about cycling that gets into your blood. I just felt good about being back on my bike and to do well was a bonus really.

'I think that night where I nearly died was what helped more than anything else. Every day that I got on my bike or went to the gym, or was on my ergonometer I had no doubt in my mind that I could push myself hard. I told myself that it would never be as hard as that day in hospital. I knew nothing could be harder and I used that every single day.'

Memories of that night never overwhelmed him. They were there in the back of his mind as the pain of over-exertion kicked in. When his lungs were burning and his legs were almost rigid with lactic acid, he would feel the phantom tubes in his nose, see the bedside nurse and then drive himself on.

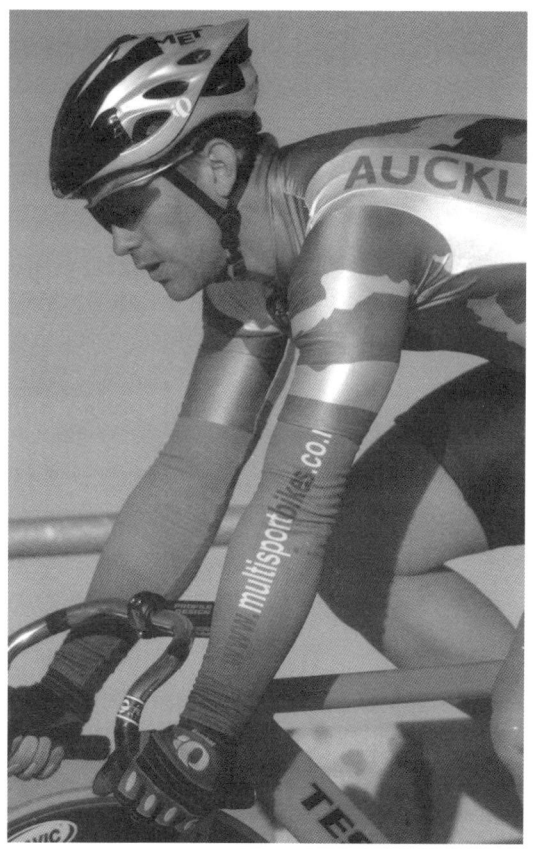

Justin Grace readies himself before winning the New Zealand Sprint title in Mosgiel, 2003.

Fears that his body would go into meltdown were beginning to subside. He wasn't complacent, far from it. He had matured. No longer did he feel he had to conform to the hard man cycling stereotype. Others could goad him at training, but if he didn't feel quite right, the verbals would fall on deaf ears. Grace was big enough to get off his bike and go home whenever his body started giving him signals.

Nor was there any residual bitterness eating away at his soul. There was no wallowing in self-pity. His hand had been dealt, and cruel bitch that fate was, nothing could be done to reverse things. There was no point in wishing he'd never had ulcerative colitis.

'I really tried not to think about it. I would always have people coming up to me and saying, "Imagine if you were well. You could do 10.4 seconds now." But I would say, "I'm not well and this is as good as I can do." I would sometimes think it would be great to be in the top three at a World Cup event rather than the top 10. But I just had to accept these were the cards I was dealt and I couldn't do anything about it.

'In the earlier days I felt I had to prove I could do what everyone else could do and of course I ended up getting sicker. At a 12-day training camp I might get to day eight or nine. Now I am that much more mature I don't feel I have got anything to prove to anyone but myself. I know that

I can get away with doing half to two-thirds the training everyone else is doing. In the early days I couldn't come to terms with that. I felt I would be at a disadvantage if I couldn't do it. We had a hard coach and I didn't feel I could ask for a day off training and I felt the rest of the team would think I was soft. In actual fact I was giving myself a huge disadvantage by doing the training. I knew that but I felt it was more important to match everyone with effort even if it meant crashing early. Now, there are some days I can push myself as hard as anyone else, while others I do my warm-up and decide to go home.'

Grace was a man whose only burden of expectation was his own. It suited him. In March 2002 he competed at the national track championships for the first time since 1993, and won the sprint silver behind Anthony Peden. More success came a month later at the Australian national championships and a fortnight later he qualified sixth fastest in a Sydney World Cup field that featured world champion, Frenchman Arnaud Tournant, and Commonwealth Games gold medal favourite Sean Eadie of Australia. Erika knew by then her husband was not being ridiculous. His dream, which had lain cold on the slab for seven years, had come back to life.

The Manchester Games started in July. He was in the form of his life. There wasn't time to ponder the insanity of the situation. In the space of a few months, Grace had done so much, worked so hard and ridden so well that it would have been heart-breaking to have missed out on selection. It seemed as if his brush with death had purpose after all. That struggle in the early hours of the morning hadn't just been about survival. It was about providing him with the tools to achieve the dreams he had always harboured. It took a while for that realisation to be made. That made it all the sweeter when the day came that his name was read out as part of the New Zealand cycling team for the Commonwealth Games.

'I had an inkling I was going to be in because there were a few phone calls asking me theoretical questions about where I would like to train if I made the team and when could I make myself available. I was at work and I kept expecting to get a phone call. We were sitting in the cafeteria having lunch when one of the guys I worked with walked past me and said congratulations. He told me he had heard on the news that I was in the team and I thought, "Oh my God, is this for real?"'

It was very much for real. Grace was a member of a sprint team that travelled to Manchester with an outside chance of a medal. Not that he was too bothered about all that. Just being there largely fulfilled his dream. He was going to be in Manchester to give of his best and have some fun. His father was coming over, too. He'd invested thousands of hours of emotion over the years. He was a shareholder in his son's dream and he wanted to be there to see this most unlikely journey arrive at a destination everyone said was impossible to reach.

'No one in New Zealand ever realised how hard things had been for Justin. I remember one rider looking at him and saying that's what happens when you take drugs. Justin was going to clout him. But people didn't understand how serious his illness was.

'After his operations I never thought he'd get back into it. I never thought he'd get back into racing so competitively. I never discouraged him, but at the back of my mind I was thinking, "What is this silly boy getting himself into now?" As a parent there is not a lot you can do. He wouldn't have listened. So I went to Manchester and that was fantastic. A really proud moment.'

Grace won a 200 metre sprint in Edinburgh shortly before the Games. But then 12 days out, disaster threatened to strike. He contracted a virus and was in bed for a few days. After all he had been through, a virus was never going to stop him. He didn't panic and, within a few days, was back on his bike.

When the time came, the goal was to beat Canada in the team sprint and get into the top five. Grace had already finished ninth in both his individual pursuits, placings that left him thrilled.

The team broke the national record three times along the way to finish fourth.

Normally, fourth is the dreaded placing of all athletes. The heartbreaking finish just outside the medals. For Grace, it was magic.

'We went there trying to get into the top five. It was going to be a hard battle. We figured we were going to be fighting Canada for fifth and sixth.

We rode three New Zealand records. We finished fourth. We were nervous as hell as we knew if something went wrong with one of the other teams we were going home with a medal. That was blowing us away.

'It was only after the games that we thought how close we were. For us to be there fighting against England, Scotland and Australia was huge. In my individual events I just wanted to ride better than I ever had. All I ever want to do is ride my best.'

And there is not a soul who could say he has fallen short on that particular goal. It is beyond dispute that riding his best is all Grace has ever done.

Justin Grace recorded the fastest sprint time for a New Zealand cyclist in August 2002, when he travelled 200 metres in 10.261 seconds. The achievement came after he took fourth place at the Manchester Commonwealth Games as part of the New Zealand sprint cycling team. He came ninth in both the individual sprint and one kilometre time trial at Manchester. He has also won nine national sprint titles between 1988 and 2006. In January 2006, at the age of 35, he was selected again to cycle for New Zealand at the Commonwealth Games in Melbourne, where he once more finished just outside the medals. He owns a bicycle shop in Newmarket, Auckland – a business he runs with his wife. He has a daughter, Cadence.

3

KELLY EVERNDEN

Davis Cup Tennis Player and ATP Tour Member 1985-1997

Kelly Evernden was not the type who was ever going to fit neatly into a box. He and convention never saw eye-to-eye. He grew up on benefits in Gisborne. It was some way removed from the stereotypical upbringing Tennis New Zealand had in mind for its budding superstars. They weren't sure quite what to make of this talented kid from a very modest broken home. Unlike many of his elite peer group, Evernden didn't experience a leisurely introduction to tennis through Mummy and Daddy's club. The family didn't enjoy a few sets and then a poolside lunch on Sunday afternoons. He fell outside the square as far as the sport's administrators were concerned.

And Evernden certainly wasn't going to be comfortable in the box that loomed as his permanent residence when he was hit by a car as a 16-year-old, rushed to hospital and pronounced dead on arrival.

Evernden was very much his own man. Strong enough to follow his heart and not worry what others thought. His peer group played rugby. He took a stand and decided tennis, no matter its perception as a sissy sport, was the game for him. It wasn't that he had set his sights on being anti-establishment. There was no grand plan to be different because he thought it might be cool. He knew what he wanted and what he liked. It helped that he came into this world equipped with an indomitable spirit. It meant he was never going to be pushed off-course. And, goodness knows, there were some fairly extreme assaults that tried to rob him of his ambition and break his soul.

Although his upbringing was underpinned by the love of a strong and doting mother, it was tough. Benefits don't allow a family budget to stretch any further than the basics. There certainly wasn't cash for tennis lessons or state-of-the-art equipment. He lived close to the bones of his backside. The whole family did once they returned to Gisborne when Evernden was 14.

There had been a five-year dalliance with Australia. The family emigrated when Evernden was nine, but divorce brought his mother, Yvonne Anne Rare, and her three offspring back to the whanau. His father only hovered on the edge of the scene and Gisborne in the mid-1970s had an uncanny ability to misguide its youth. It wasn't New Zealand's top corporations that came trying to recruit from Gisborne's schools. Life's less savoury and illicit operators held more sway, offering careers on the wrong side of the law. When all the facts were weighed up, Evernden seemed not to have the remotest chance of finding a pathway that would lead him to Wimbledon's hallowed turf.

That was never going to stop him succeeding, though. The fact he would be starting his journey from left field simply meant his route to the pinnacle of the game would have to be circuitous. Then again, that was nothing new as his motivation for taking up tennis was a touch unusual. Evernden loved the sport for the one-on-one confrontation it afforded. While in Australia he had boxed. The noble art had instilled a passion for combat – both physical and mental. Tennis was a game where he felt he could let out the mongrel. For most other young New Zealanders, rugby was the vehicle used to jettison copious testosterone. But Evernden didn't feel rugby was going to soak up all his competitive juices. As he says: 'I had an experience with rugby that made me think, "You know what, I want to do something on my own," so I was the guy to blame. I was told literally by the coach I was the reason we lost the game. I looked at him and said, "Okay. That's a good thing to tell a kid. That's a good healthy approach."

I decided I was pretty good at tennis and if I lost then I knew I lost because of me. I like that individual thing better.

'I don't mind taking the blame when I'm wrong, but I hate taking the blame when I'm right. I don't think it was that difficult for me. I boxed a lot before I came back from Australia and I think tennis has a similar mentality. You know people look at it as a sissy sport but that one-on-one pugilistic aspect of it always appealed to me. I am a fairly aggressive person and playing tennis suited my personality quite well.

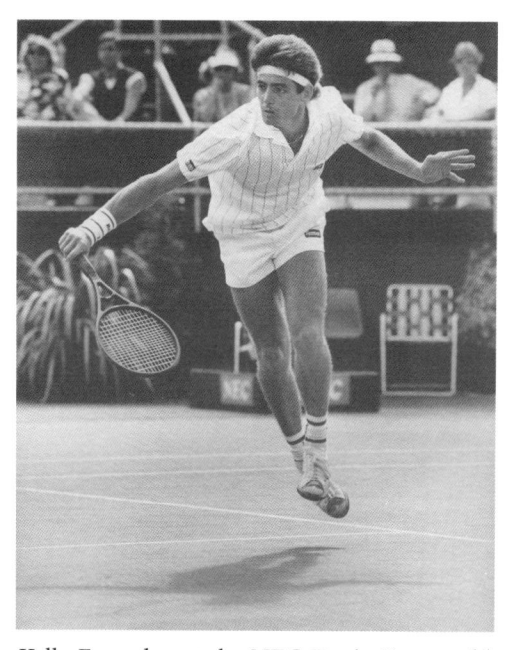

Kelly Evernden at the NEC Davis Cup world group contest at Stanley Street, March 1986. *New Zealand Herald*

'I guess it suited me because I had a pretty tough upbringing. We went to a lot of different high schools and you know what that is like. I didn't have a lot of backing. Being the oldest son a lot fell on me so it made me a little tougher than perhaps I should have been.'

He was tough all right. He was tough enough to win the New Zealand National Under-16 title. He was tough enough to persuade Tennis New Zealand that while he didn't fit the stereotype, he had a game and attitude that was worth investing in. He was tough enough to survive being run over – an accident that led to him being revived by electric shock therapy, losing his right lung, smashing his left leg and separating his left elbow from the rest of his arm. But most importantly, he was tough enough to never stop believing in himself when he came out of hospital.

Others would also have shown the necessary will to live and survive the crash. But Evernden didn't just survive. He went on to enjoy 13 years on the ATP tour, winning three tournaments, and he was New Zealand's

Davis Cup saviour more times than he can remember. He even beat John McEnroe. The odds of him achieving so much on the professional tennis circuit would have been around a million to one against – maybe higher – when at the tender age of 16 he arrived at Gisborne Hospital in a state of quite considerable disrepair.

'I was one of the top players in New Zealand. I had won the New Zealand Under-16 national title the year before against Rob Lewis. I was definitely one of the guys they were earmarking for whatever was going to happen in New Zealand tennis. But I got run over. We were at a bowling hall out at Makaraka. It was a teenage party kind of thing. I was probably being a bit stupid. We were leaving the party and the next thing I know I woke up a couple of weeks later in hospital. I was getting into my friend's car, holding on to the door handle when a car coming the other way hit me.

'He stopped. I knew the guy. I went to school with him but I can't remember his name. It was definitely not his fault. It was probably my fault. I was standing in the dark, getting into a car and should have been paying a bit more attention. The wing mirror of the car did most of the damage. It took my right lung out and broke all my ribs. The day before my friend had filed the wing mirror of his car down. It had been at a rough point and he filed about an inch and a half off. If he hadn't done that, I would not be here.

'Apparently when I arrived my mother was in a police car coming to hospital and she heard over the radio there was a "Dead on Arrival" at the hospital. That's why they had the paddles. I was in the intensive care unit for about 10 days and then I was moved into the main ward. I think when I first woke up I was in shock. I didn't know what had happened and I woke up expecting to go to school. I remember looking at myself in the roof because it was all mirrors and I thought, "Who is that guy lying there?" I was kind of on the verge of waking up and I was looking at this guy with tubes going everywhere and casts all over his body and thinking, "Oh my God!"

'All of a sudden I realised it was me. Then the doctors came in and said, "Nice of you to join us." I never got the feeling from them that they were surprised that I had woken up. I think one of the greatest experiences of my life was the nursing staff and doctors in that hospital. I never felt defeated. They never said, "You shouldn't have made it," or, "You are going to be a cripple." I think a large part of the positive attitude I adopted was due to them. They were phenomenal.'

But just because Evernden's heart was once again beating, the odds on him making it to the professional circuit didn't shorten. If anything, they lengthened. Most elite athletes boast a full complement of vital organs. Evernden was only going to be taking one lung out of the hospital with him. And his left leg was only doing its job courtesy of a 17-inch steel pin. If he'd been a racehorse, he wouldn't have been going home from the hospital. He would have been off to the glue factory.

It wasn't just his reduced physical capacity that was counting against him. Tennis New Zealand, who weren't exactly clutching Evernden to their bosom prior to the accident, let their tenuous grip slip altogether. The maverick from Gisborne had proved their reservations to be well founded. They had suspected Evernden would only go and prove them right to be dubious about his ability to last the distance. Clearly, with just the one lung and a leg that would set off metal detectors at airports, Evernden was best tossed on the scrap heap.

'When you lose a lung, you have to wonder how it is going to affect you. At that age you wonder whether you are going to be the guy on oxygen when you are 40. I didn't have enough knowledge to know how big an effect the loss of my lung was going to have on me.

'The leg issue, in my mind, was something that was just broken. I had seen kids with broken legs before so I thought I would be fine. The arm was a bit of an issue because it was separated at the elbow and they said I would only have 40 per cent mobility. That was actually quite good because it gave me something to do when I was in hospital. I had a handle above my bed. I spent all day hanging on it with my left arm because I wanted it to straighten out. To this day I don't sleep very much – maybe five or six hours a day. So having so much forced bedtime, you have to find things to do. Tedious kinds of things that were physically necessary, I did them all day long. I actually got my arm past straight, so I guess I overdid it. It now extends more than my right arm.

'The leg was shattered and with the arm on the same side it was impossible for me to use crutches. I went home in a wheelchair and when they thought the arm was strong enough they let me use crutches. I used to walk in the shower and I thought the leg was pretty good. I was out of the wheelchair as soon as I got home. My mum was pretty mad at me but the leg turned out to be stronger than the doctors thought.

'But when the accident happened, Tennis New Zealand took the view, "Oh well, he's done, we can write him off." It didn't really bother me. My mother had more conversations with them than I did. I think they still looked at me as this rebellious kid who was outside the mainstream of where they expected tennis players to come from. I didn't come from Auckland, from a wealthy family, and I have a bit of attitude. I had a lot of talent but I think they viewed me as a wild card. My mother got pissed off and said, "We will do it our way." She was angrier than I was.

'Maybe she had a lack of understanding about what they were trying to do with me at that stage. Maybe she had a greater commitment to me than I had to me at that stage. My mother was the reason that things got back on track and back together. A lot of the reasons I kept going were down to her determination.'

Instilled with his mother's confidence, love and support, Evernden slipped back into civilian life. He had been in hospital for six months following his accident. He didn't want to make a hero's return. He simply wanted to assimilate and begin his life where he left off. Normality was his objective. And normality meant getting back on to the tennis court. That's where he spent much of his time pre-accident. Despite his obvious talent and early success, he had no pre-accident visions of himself one day travelling the world as a tournament pro. Tennis was recreation for Evernden. It was what he did instead of putting on a scrum-cap and smashing into people. His desire to get back on the court was not about rekindling broken dreams. It was about bringing routine and structure back to his life.

Except there was one mighty problem – he could barely get out of his chair without having to gasp for breath and start sucking the oxygen as if it was soon to be rationed. His left lung had not been consulted about the new working practices. It had been quite happily working in tandem with its partner, only to have its workload doubled with no significant warning. There was no point talking to the union rep about matters. Evernden, as the boss, was going to have to get his one lung doing the work of two. It wasn't something open for debate. There was no alternative, as a transplant lung was not an option. Regardless of the burning pain, regardless of the oxygen debt and lactic acid build-up, Evernden was going to have to persevere. He was going to have to put his breathing organ through the sort of boot camp that only the SAS of the lung world would survive.

'At that stage I don't think I had a vision that I was good enough or there was even the prospect of being able to play tennis for a living. It never occurred to me. It wasn't until I was a junior in college and the agents started turning up on my doorstep offering me money that I realised this was something I could do as a career. It was a slow awakening for me. I wasn't one of those kids who were groomed to be a gifted athlete from early in life.

'I started playing tennis not too long after I got home. But I was playing gingerly and slowly. The big thing for me was building up my wind. I couldn't walk more than 100 metres without getting winded because of my lung. I started running on the beach. Once I got to the point where I thought I could play a little bit, I built my endurance.

'Initially I didn't think I was ever going to be able to run again. The scar tissue in the remaining lung was so decompressed. I would run 100 metres and I was gasping.

'Previously, I could run five miles no problem. So I would pack a lunch and run and stop. Run and stop. I would end up 10 miles away from home and then I would turn around and then run and stop and run and stop until I got back home. It would sometimes take me four or five hours but that was the only way I could force myself to keep going. If I had just run around the block I would have got tired and then come home.

'When I moved to Wellington a couple of years later, I was getting a bit fitter. I would run up and down the firebreaks in the hills round Lower Hutt. I think that was the turning point as far as my breathing and stamina were concerned. That was a real grind. I was in these firebreaks

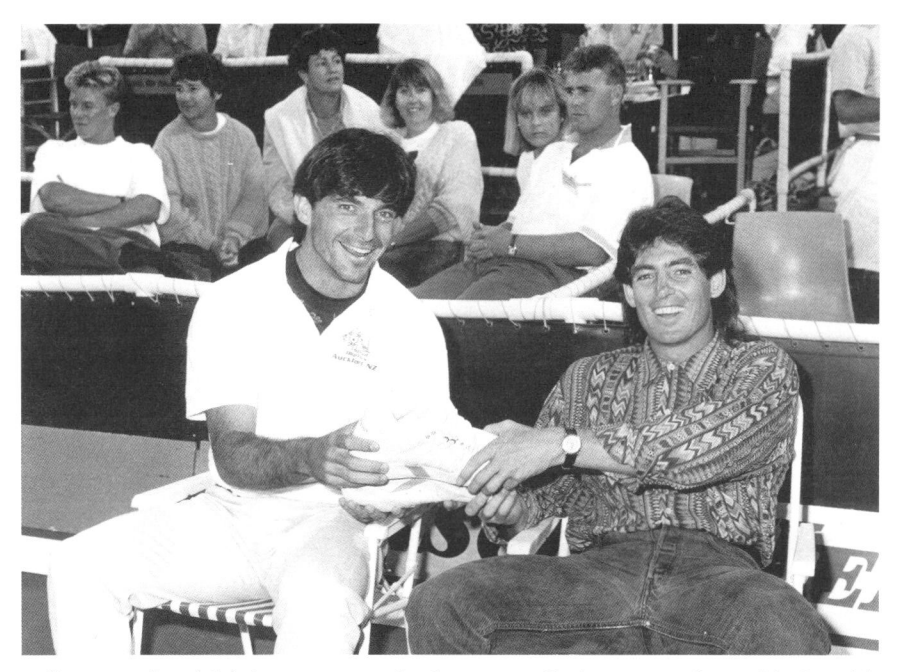

Kelly Evernden (right) uses a tennis shoe as a Christmas cracker with Spanish professional Emilio Sanchez at the 1991 Heineken Open in Auckland. *Auckland Tennis*

and I was walking halfway and running halfway. A few months later and I was running all the way up. I felt like I had really accomplished something. From that point on, I never looked at the lungs as a liability.'

His leg, though, was a different story. He was getting by on the court. Playing at a decent level, but he was not quite the force he once was. It was his speed – it had been greatly reduced by the accident. He couldn't chase and scamper the way he did of old. His game was built on aggression. He harried opponents with his energy and determination. That was proving kind of hard with a hunk of metal sticking out of his hip.

Given that Evernden had survived 10 days in intensive care, six months in hospital and almost a year of physical torture recovering his stamina, his leg wasn't going to be an insurmountable problem. His mother had taken care of some of his other problems by sending him away from Gisborne. A family friend from Australia managed to squeeze Evernden into a college in the States and it was there that he would finish his schooling. Evernden's mother had never stopped believing her son would take his place among the game's elite. The lack of support from Tennis New Zealand only made her more determined. She knew that if she could get her son away from Gisborne, where there were too many negative influences, she could get his faith in himself up to the levels she possessed.

'If I had goals in life, Gisborne wasn't really the place that would help me fulfil them. I don't think being marked at 16 is unique in New Zealand. I don't know if that is the reason she wanted me out of there. The environment wasn't right. There wasn't a lot of promise for me if I stayed around and wallowed in self-pity. She didn't let me get into that downward spiral. Not that I felt I was likely to get into one. The accident was just something that happened. I never looked at it and thought, "Why couldn't this have happened to someone else?" I thought, "Wow, let's see what we can do from here and try not to let this happen again."

'I went to Yakima Valley Community College in Washington State. That was the beginning of the next phase. I had all these pins in my body and plates and I didn't play as well as I could. A friend of ours knew an orthopaedic surgeon and he wanted to have a look at my leg. The pin in my left leg was causing me a lot of pain and discomfort because it was actually sticking out of my hip. He went in and looked at it and said he didn't think I needed it so he took it out. That was the turning point for my game.

'I was always extremely fast and the pin made me very ordinary on the tennis court as far as speed goes. As soon as he took the pin out I went from doing okay, but kind of battling, to all of a sudden having the speed to match my vision on the court. Then it was exciting. My stamina was great.'

It was exciting all right. A scholarship to Arkansas University put him in rarefied company. His game was being exposed to the best young players in the world. His name was being touted by agents who were all keen to sign him up and take him to the lucrative ATP circuit. The bigtime was a real possibility. And yet, never once did Evernden stop to think about how far he had come. Those six months in hospital in Gisborne never flashed into his mind as he took the court. He didn't win a game and then think it all the sweeter for having done so with just one lung. That wasn't his way. And for good reason, too. His focus was not on the past. He couldn't afford to be soft on himself. He didn't want to think of himself as an exceptional athlete with one lung. He wanted to be an exceptional athlete. Full stop. No sympathy or allowances to be made. Few things in life raised his hackles higher than having famous victories become all about a car accident he was involved in as a 16-year-old. He wanted to be acknowledged for his all-round game, not his ability to survive 10 days in a coma.

'By the time I went to the University of Arkansas, I had established myself as a really good tennis player. I guess if you are an astronaut and you have one lung they are going to look at your past. But if you are still beating the people in your peer group, I think that speaks more than past injuries. My lung was never an issue for anyone at Arkansas. They never asked me about it or had any reservations about taking me on a scholarship. I played there for four years and then went on to the pro tour.

'I never really thought about my accident. I always looked at it as something people could pick on. I thought people would make something of the fact there was this kid who grew up on welfare in Gisborne playing professional tennis with Boris Becker and John McEnroe. If I came in there and said, "I have only got one lung," then maybe they were not going to appreciate the fact that I was doing what I was doing pretty well. I never came off and said, "I just beat John McEnroe and I only have one lung." I used to get quite angry with that.

'I can remember beating Michael Chang in the quarter-finals of a tournament in San Francisco. I beat him pretty badly and he was number three in the world at the time. I came off the court and was being interviewed and the guy said, "You know you only have one lung?" Like I didn't know that I only have one lung. I was looking at him and thinking, "How fucking stupid are you?" I know I only have one lung but it's not as if I wake up every morning and count them. It was kind of sad because the viewers from then on thought about this guy with one lung beating

Michael Chang. That was mainly the reason I never really talked about it because it took over from the fact I had played one of the best matches of my life.

'I guess I never wanted to feel I had overachieved. When you are trying to be as good as you can any excuse will tip you over. If I started thinking I shouldn't be this good because I only have one lung, suddenly I might not be as competitive. I am not sure that is the reason or maybe you realise there is no place for it. You have got a new endeavour and you have to put all the things that are distractions out of the way.'

One of those distractions was his relationship with Tennis New Zealand. Once Evernden was established on the ATP tour, he became the obvious man to lead New Zealand's Davis Cup team. That could have been problematic. But Evernden wasn't going to hold a grudge. What would be the point? He was realistic enough to appreciate that a few days after his accident, he really didn't look like a potential Davis Cup player. He backed himself as did his mother, but it was going to be a hard, probably impossible, sell, convincing others to retain their faith.

'I have a great relationship with the guys who were running New Zealand tennis while I was there. Talking to them as an adult, you bury it. I was the only person ranked high enough to lead the team so I looked at it as a chance to show how good I was. I could have said, "No, you were mean to me and my mother," but I thought if I am the guy you are betting on I am going to try and be a pretty good horse.'

The list of achievements is proof indeed that Evernden was a more than useful horse. In his 13 years as a professional, he won three singles tournaments and five doubles tournaments on the ATP tour. He was New Zealand Residential champion four times and played 20 Davis Cup ties. He finished his professional career with 135 wins and 146 losses. His personal highlight was making the quarterfinals of the Australian Open in 1987. It was made all the more special by the fact his mother was in Melbourne.

The 1990 Davis Cup win against Yugoslavia in Christchurch is another personal highlight, as was defeating McEnroe. At his peak Evernden had a world ranking of 31, a figure no Kiwi in the last 10 years has come remotely close to emulating. It is a record that stands him alongside the very best New Zealand has ever produced. The astonishing thing is, though, that his former coach, Jeff Simpson, believes that Evernden could have been even better. The boy from Gisborne perhaps got a little too hung-up about being the boy from Gisborne and lacked a little self-belief when he first started keeping company with the biggest names. There was a sense of awe that took a while to overcome.

'What he went through obviously gave him a fair amount of determination and strength,' says Simpson. 'You can't come through something like that and not have those characteristics. He had more talent in his little toe than most of us have in our whole bodies. But he'll be the first to admit he wasn't always as focused as he could have been when he first went on the circuit. It is hard to make it as a professional in any sport. Kelly never imagined that someone from his background, from an out of the way place like New Zealand, could ever make it. My job was really about getting him to focus on being a professional both on and off the court. That was the big challenge for Kelly. It took him a while to believe in himself and focus on what he wanted to achieve but once he did that, he had that killer instinct.

'I can't remember Kelly ever mentioning his lung while he was playing. When he was playing in the Davis Cup team it never impeded him. He would get so wound up in those matches that he would play in the singles and doubles back-to-back but he never lacked stamina. He didn't want people to talk about his lung or accident. He was worried opponents would perceive him as weak.

'He probably could have gone further than 31 in the world. He had the ability. But you have to say his was an amazing achievement. When you think how far he came and what he went through. He won three ATP tour events and played so many Davis Cup games.'

It took Evernden some time to come round to Simpson's way of thinking. It's not as if he now punctuates his time coaching in the US by wallowing in a self-congratulatory mire. Far from it. His accident and professional tennis career are both behind him and he is not the sort of guy who gets a big kick out of gazing into the rearview mirror. But there have been occasions, however, when he has glanced back to his previous life and felt the first warm rising of pride.

'I was a little bit starstruck when I first started. Walking into the locker room at Wimbledon was intimidating. But I realised I had to make these guys believe I could compete with them. I don't think there is anything more satisfying than going one-on-one with someone who everyone else thinks is far superior physically and mentally and coming out on top. That is the underdog attitude I have had my whole life. I was the underdog no matter what the odds were.

'I had a few moments of reminiscing after I stopped playing. I played some great Davis Cup matches in New Zealand. We beat Yugoslavia in Christchurch and I remember sitting there after, thinking, "That's a pretty far place to come for a guy who was lying on a gurney in hospital." I appreciate that now more than I ever did when I was younger. I don't know if I was worried about it becoming a distraction or if I was worried about it taking away the focus from what I was doing. But I have sat back since then and thought I have done well.'

There wouldn't be a chorus of dissent if Evernden broke character one day and claimed that he had maybe even done very well.

Kelly Evernden remains one of New Zealand's most successful Davis Cup representatives. He played in 20 ties, winning 17 and losing 17 singles matches and winning 10 and losing 10 doubles encounters. He is also the only New Zealander to have won on the ATP professional circuit, when he was victorious in Bristol, Brisbane and Wellington. In a career that saw him cross paths with many of the game's greats such as John McEnroe, Pete Sampras, Boris Becker and Stefan Edberg, Evernden won almost US$1 million in prize money. After he retired from the professional circuit he went on to coach and he is currently the club professional at Mercer Island Country Club in Seattle, Washington.

4

BRADLEY ILES
Professional Golfer 2005–

Everything was as it should have been in the Iles household on 18 July 2004. Peter and Karen Iles were parked in front of the box in their Papamoa home. They were watching *Close Up at Seven*, engrossed in a story about floods in Waimana, when the phone rang. Karen answered. She identified herself, listened for a few seconds and then her quivering hand passed the receiver to her husband.

What Peter Iles heard was an American voice asking him if he was the father of a Bradley Iles. When he answered, 'Yes,' Peter learned that his son was unconscious after sustaining a major head trauma. The caller said to stay by the phone. Iles ended the call, too shocked to take on board what he had just heard.

It only took a couple of minutes before the device was filling the room with its shrill tones again. Iles said 'Hello' and heard the caller introduce himself as a surgeon at the University Memorial Hospital in Savannah, Georgia. The doctor explained that they needed to get Bradley into the operating theatre immediately. It was a matter of life and death. There was blood pumping out of his young patient's head. He reckoned that Bradley maybe had about four hours to live. Probably two had already been taken up getting to hospital and tracking down his parents on

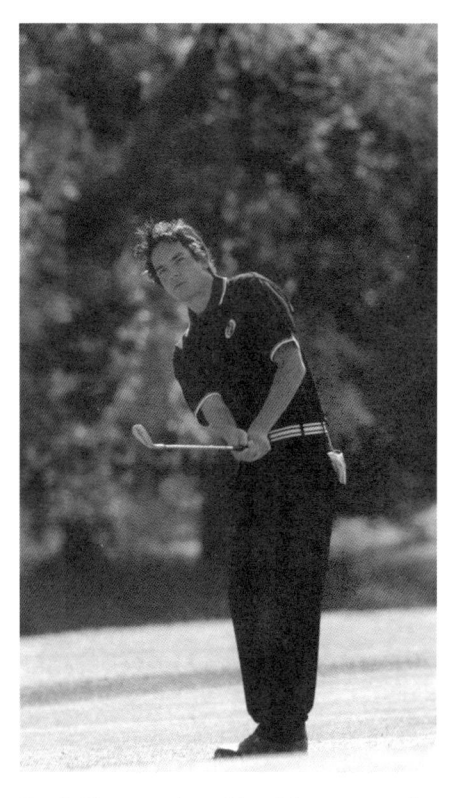

Brad Iles watches his chip on to the green at the Asia Pacific Amateur Championship in Japan, 2005.

the other side of the world. The surgeon wanted permission to begin the procedure. 'Of course,' trembled the crackly voice at the other end.

It was the call every parent desperately hopes they will never have to field. Peter hung up. And then he and his wife were consumed by the most terrifying helplessness. Their precious son, still only 20, was lying unconscious in a foreign land. He maybe only had a few hours to live. The surgeon had stressed the gravity of the situation. 'You must understand, Mr Iles,' he said, 'if we don't operate, your son will die.' The house had never been so quiet. What could either of them say? They couldn't offer reassurance. Neither of them could confidently declare their son was going to be okay. They had no idea. They barely even knew how it was he came to be bleeding so profusely in the first place. They sat in mental torment waiting for some kind of update. When the phone rang a couple of hours later, neither Peter nor Karen was sure whether they wanted to answer it.

Prior to the first call from the hospital, the last report they had of their son had been of a more positive nature. Bradley was one of New Zealand's most talented young golfers. He had been part of the Rotorua Boys' High School team that had won the world schools' championship in 2001. By 2003 he was winning New Zealand's biggest amateur events and in the same year he reached the final of Australia's national championship. Young Iles had the talent to make a big name for himself. The professional ranks loomed. The grand plan was to spend the summer of 2004 in the States where he would have a couple of months playing in golf's biggest amateur events. If he could survive over there, he knew he would be ready to turn pro at the end of the year. His venture had gone well. He won a tournament in Canada. Made it to the final of another in the US where he lost in a play-off and then, at the Players Amateur in South Carolina, he finished a superb ninth. This was recognised as one of the biggest amateur tournaments outside the majors. Iles was blown away by his performance at the Belfair Golf Club.

His parents would have been too, but they had no idea he had done so well. All they knew was that the phone was ringing and one of them needed to answer it. Peter lifted the receiver.

'It was the surgeon. He told us the surgery had been fine and they had Brad in an induced coma and he had settled down. Karen is a nurse and she knows about these kinds of things. They had put a device in Brad's head to measure the pressure of the brain. Karen rang every hour after that. The pressure rose for a while during the night and we were getting quite concerned. We didn't get any sleep.

'The next day there was a flight to Los Angeles at four pm. We had no idea what had been happening on this 13-hour flight. Before we had got on the plane we had been in touch all the time. We were sitting on the plane and halfway across Karen said, "One way or another we are going to get our son home." We didn't know. We thought he might not have made it.'

If there was a worse way to spend 13 hours neither Karen nor Peter could think of one. They crossed the Pacific with heavy hearts. This was most definitely a trip they did not want to be making. As they made their descent into Los Angeles Airport they tried to somehow make sense of the dramatic twist their lives had taken since the hospital first phoned. Brad was in the States playing golf – a sport with an established and long history of sending its participants home in one piece. How could things have gone so badly wrong? Who was responsible for this terrible mess? Karen and Peter were afforded little solace when they found out that, in an indirect way, alligators were to blame.

Bradley's memory is hazy but he can recall that a few hours after he had walked off the 18th green at the Players, he and a few Australian players went back to the house where they were all staying and blew the froth off a few cold ones. Once a few had slipped down, Iles and his chums felt the overwhelming desire to go and find some alligators.

'We just wanted to check them out,' says Iles. 'See what they were up to. They come up to the road quite a lot. I can't really remember that night. I just know what other people have told me. We were in a private resort called Belfair in Hilton Head, South Carolina. It was a big complex and gated so no one could get in or out. Everyone got around on golf carts and they were pretty damned fast. They could get up to 50 km/h.

'I jumped on the back of a cart and Anthony Brown and Gavin Flint [Australian golfers] were in the front. We were on the road and there was a path that went off to the left and a path that went off to the right. I thought we were going to the left, so I lent to the left. We were going pretty fast. But we went right. I cracked the right side of my head. I think I must have had something in my right hand – maybe a can of Budweiser – so I was hanging on with my left hand. We went right, I spun off and my whole body just went. It took them a while to realise I had fallen off. When they came back for me I was lying on my back on the road and I was in a pool of blood that was bigger than my body. If you imagine that I was lying like an angel in the sand with my arms right out, then the blood went out further than my arms and legs. One of the guys spewed when he saw me. He couldn't handle it.

'Anthony Brown got underneath my head and pulled me back on to him. He said I was trying to get up and run around. I was in a terrible state. I couldn't speak. Anthony was holding me back. Aaron Price [another Australian golfer travelling in a different cart] took his shirt off and tried to put some pressure on my head. The blood was spraying out everywhere because I had burst an artery. I had a hat on and it was black and white. They thought it was a red hat. My jeans were soaked in blood. Aaron rang 911 and got the ambulance to come.

'He said the ambulance drivers were hopeless. He said they didn't even care. They picked me up and threw me in the back of the van. He was yelling at them. At that stage they didn't realise how bad I was. It was only when we were driving that they realised the situation was serious so they changed plans on the way and took me to the University Memorial Hospital. That was where there were neurological surgeons.'

And that was where Iles's life was saved. When his parents called from Los Angeles for a progress report they learned that the doctors had turned off the life support machine and Iles had continued to breathe unaided. It was a good sign. Death had retreated to the shadows but there was still huge uncertainty as to how much damage had been done. The brain had taken a massive blow. The concussion was severe and the bleeding had been allowed to continue for longer than the doctors would have liked. The ambulance had been delayed trying to get into Belfair and then it had taken time to track down a number for Peter and Karen to gain their permission to begin operating. It was after 11 pm when Karen and Peter arrived in Savannah – it straddles the border between Georgia and South Carolina – and they really had no idea what to expect.

'When we phoned the hospital from LA, they said they would try to wake Brad when we arrived,' recalls Peter. 'He opened his eyes and said, "Hello," but then he closed his eyes and disappeared again. He did seem to recognise us. He was like that for the next five or six days. They were trying to keep him alert.

'The doctors were saying the whole time that they didn't know what was going to happen. It could get worse or it could get better. Brain traumas take a long time to recover from. They were trying to prepare us for the worst and keep our hopes down.'

It wasn't necessarily a difficult battle for the doctors. Peter and Karen did not arrive in the States with big expectations. They desperately wanted their son to make a full recovery but they had braced themselves for the worst. With Brad now drifting in and out of consciousness, they felt they were almost in bonus territory. Over the next few days Brad fell into a pattern where he would come to, show some faint recognition of his parents and then return to his comatose state.

The doctors were happy. They felt it was only a matter of time before Brad would stop drifting. Peter and Karen were feeling more confident.

Their worst fears had subsided a little. It was still going to be a very long road back for Brad. It was still possible that he might have reduced faculties or limited physical ability. But they could only cross those bridges if they ever came to them. Their focus was on the very short term and they were encouraged by the fact Brad continued to stay awake for longer periods each day. Then, just as a little sunshine appeared to be creeping into their lives, some very threatening rain-clouds gathered.

Brad had a bad night eight days after his accident. He'd been found wandering around the hospital. He was returned to his bed and handcuffed to it. Somehow he managed to persuade one of the nurses that the cuffs were cutting into him so she agreed to take them off. Brad took his chance and immediately went walkabout again. When Peter and Karen arrived the next morning they felt decidedly uneasy.

'We got to the hospital and Brad was dozy,' is Peter's recollection. 'The doctor who had done the surgery came in and we said we were concerned about Brad – we said, "He doesn't seem to be getting anywhere." So he said he would take a look at the pictures of Brad's brain. He did that and then said, "Yes, it is getting worse. It looks like his brain is swelling and we might have to go in and do more surgery." That was even more terrifying. He went and had a consultation with a lot of other doctors and after that he came back and gave Brad a super dose of whatever drugs they were giving him. He said, "Come back in two hours." We were feeling awful so we went for a walk. We were wondering what he was going to be like and we were worried that they were going to have to do more surgery. But when we got to his room, there he was sitting up in bed eating ice-cream – the little bugger. He looked at us and said, "Mum, Dad, what are you doing here?" It was the first time he had properly recognised us.'

The relief flowed through Peter and Karen like a good wine. They had come to America to get their boy – one way or another. He would be coming back the way they wanted. That said, though, it was still one day at a time for Brad. He had been mainly unconscious for eight days. He could hardly walk. Simple physical tasks were well beyond him. It would be a case of literally taking baby steps. The next week was spent re-learning how to walk and gradually rebuilding his strength and fine motor skills.

He lost 13 kg in the aftermath of the accident. Some fluid had seeped from his brain into his jaw and he could barely open his mouth wide enough to slide in a wafer biscuit.

He also had to contend with enormous media interest. The New Zealand media had heard about his plight and the day after his accident Iles was the lead item on TV1's sports news. The American golf-writing fraternity also picked up on the story and the hospital was flooded with TV cameras and reporters all hoping to break the latest update. It was a compelling story: a rising star of golf cut down only hours after he had enjoyed possibly the best performance of his life – one that suggested he had a serious future as a professional. The attention was welcome on one level – despite its high participation and growing global popularity golf still struggles to win its rightful share of media coverage in New Zealand.

Iles had become accustomed to seeing his efforts largely ignored while some fairly ordinary rugby players bathed in a limelight they scarcely deserved. It made a refreshing change to be the centre of attention. His profile was being raised and there would be a significantly higher number of New Zealanders now aware of the aspiring golfer Bradley Iles. But there was also a downside – he wasn't ready to cope with the demands of the press mob. Life was still a very big trial for Iles.

'There was a lot of memory loss. I got angry at the most stupid things. I can remember trying to read a book and I couldn't do it because I couldn't remember the last line I had read. I would walk around and it wouldn't feel like the real world. The brain fluid that seeped into my jaw also went into my ear and that damaged my balance. Whenever I looked down I would have pretty bad vertigo. My head would spin really badly and I would want to be sick. I really struggled with my memory, emotions and thoughts.

'It took nine days for me to fully regain consciousness. Apparently the first time I woke up my mum was at my bed and she said I didn't know who she was. I looked at her and didn't say anything. She said, "I'm your mother." And I said, "Yeah, you look like my mother but I don't think you are." I did that about eight times. I would slip into unconsciousness, wake up and say the same thing. They would tell me what happened, then I would slip under again, wake up and they would have to tell me again what happened.

'Two other people had come into the hospital at the same time with similar injuries. One came out quadriplegic and the other died. I drew the lucky straw I suppose. They didn't know what sort of trauma my brain had gone through. They knew blood supply had been taken for some time but they didn't know what damage there would be. It was about 17 days after the accident before they let me out of hospital. They were amazed at my recovery. I had to go and get an MRI scan and a hearing test. They flew me back first class because my body was so tired from lying in a bed for two-and-a-half weeks. If I was sitting up, after a few minutes, everything would start spinning and I would feel like I was going to vomit. I had to lie flat.

'When I got to Auckland I was met by all these cameras. I felt like Bruce Willis or something. There were flashes and clicking right in my face but I didn't mind it. I felt pretty good. It was tough to talk normally and remember what I was talking about. I was eager to get home.'

It had been an exhausting and traumatic few weeks for Iles and his family. On the afternoon of 17 July (USA time), Iles had been riding on one of the biggest highs of his life. Then, a few hours later he went riding on a golf cart – a journey that brought him down and delivered him alarmingly close to death. When he got back to the family home in the Bay of Plenty he tried to assess the true impact of the last few weeks. When he stripped it back to the basics he could see there was a major positive – he was still alive. And there was a major negative – he had been told that he would not be able to play golf for at least two years.

But worse still, he'd also been told that he might never be able to get back to the level he had been at. His hand-eye coordination could be permanently challenged. His brain might not be able to cope with the mental rigour of top-level golf. His concentration was very limited in the infancy of his recovery. No one could be sure it would necessarily get much better. It was a fair bet that his ninth place at the Players Amateur was going to be his 15 minutes of fame. No one doubted he would be able to recover sufficiently to play the game. No one really doubted that Iles would recover enough to once again challenge for amateur titles in New Zealand. But there seemed only an infinitesimal chance of Iles one day walking the fairways alongside the game's biggest names. The dream of playing professionally was most likely over.

Yet Iles was strangely ambivalent about his predicament. He kept golf off his daily physical and mental agenda. It wasn't that hard to do. The severity and duration of his headaches was not relenting. He was still suffering from terrible vertigo and just looking at his feet was enough to send his head spinning and his stomach churning. Then there was the chronic fatigue and memory loss. He couldn't think about golf while he was in this state. So he didn't.

'The doctors know what happens with people who have brain injuries. I thought, "Two years, who cares, it is only two years. As long as I am still upright and breathing I'll be happy with two years." I didn't really think about golf when I got back.

'The only time I did was about two days after I got home. I went to the golf course for a TV show. My dad took me there and I dropped a ball and had an eight-metre putt. I hit it really quickly, as while I was starting to think about it, my head started spinning and I couldn't really look down. I hit it straight in the hole. Dad and I looked at each other and thought, "It is still there." I had to lie down on the grass after that.

'But there would have been about two or three months where I didn't think about golf. I didn't worry about it. I had a lot of people on my side who were giving me a lot of positive reinforcement. Mal Tongue, my coach, was ringing me a lot. He came up and saw me the week after I got home. He had been talking to the doctors and they had said two years. But we said we would just see what we feel. We will go with what the body thinks it can handle.

'In September and October I used to chip a ball round the back garden for hours. I would flop balls over the corner of the house or try and make them come down the roof, jump into the gutter and then land in a bucket. It was about trying to get my imagination back. My mum and dad would come out and ask me to play certain shots and put money on it. Dad even asked me to chip balls over the bonnet of his car.

'My mind before the accident was always in the future. But during those first few months after the accident, I was living in the moment. Once I started to feel a bit stronger, by about November, I went to the gym a lot. I would pick up a weight and my arms would shake really badly. My arms would move about 10 cm and shake really quickly. I would put my hand out and it would shake. I would have little blank moments. Sometimes the whole room would shake in front of me for a few seconds. I was always tired and the drugs I was on made me tired as well.

'But it was the best thing for me. I was catching the bus to the gym and that would take about an hour. I couldn't drive and I didn't have much else to do. I did get a little bit angry that they wouldn't let me drive. Nor would they let me ride a bike, drink or swim. Not being able to do those things that I had previously taken for granted made me angrier than anything else. It was tough not being able to do simple things. But it is good to go through tough times to help put things in perspective.'

By the end of this first four months of rehabilitation Iles had no shortage of perspective. He could see now how precious his golf career was. His passion for the sport was slowly being rekindled. He was starting to think beyond chipping balls in the back garden. He knew that he didn't want to be living off his pre-accident achievements. He still felt he could be better than that. He was sure that while the accident had been traumatic, the damage was not irreversible. Iles knew that if he kept working, he'd keep improving. He thought that, in two years, he would be playing as well as he ever had.

When December ushered in some warmer weather, Iles was back out on the course, striking balls in earnest. It was just like old times, except for one major flaw – his old swing had deserted him. Understandably, he wasn't swinging the club like a potential champion any more. The timing was a little out of synch. His brain didn't have the ability to sense the rhythm any more. Which was a major problem as, almost 18 months ahead of schedule, Iles had decided he would make his competitive playing return in January 2005.

'I could pick up a club and swing it but I wouldn't know how to fix it if it was wrong. I swung like a kid would. The first shot I hit was about a

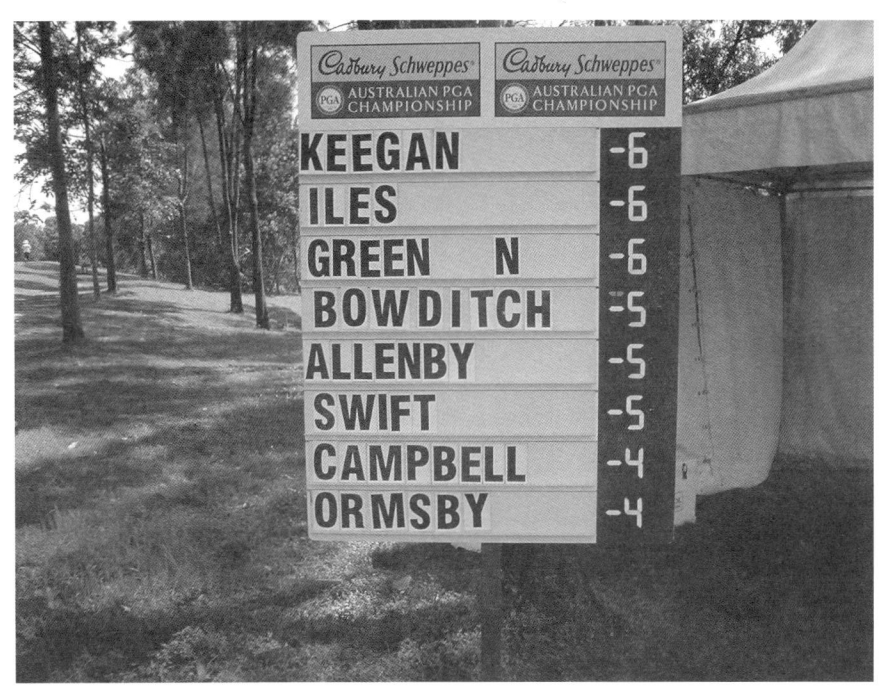

The scoreboard at the second round of the Australian PGA in 2005 shows Brad Iles' name ahead of Michael Campbell and Robert Allenby. *Peter Iles*

week after I got home. It was out in the front yard and I hit an 8-iron over the fence, over the cars, over the power lines and into the dunes that are about 120 yards from our house. I flushed it. My parents and I had a bit of a laugh, said I could maybe get back before two years, and went back in and watched the news.

'When I went to see Mal for the first time after my accident, he said I had never swung it as good as I did then. But that soon changed. Once I started hitting more balls it didn't become that natural any more. It got pretty bad pretty quick. We had to construct my swing a lot of times. I had lost that muscle memory. It went backwards really badly three times. We were planning on the New Zealand Under-23 Championship in Hastings for my comeback. All I was trying to do was make the cut. I wasn't really worrying about whether I could play well. I had a lot of time up my sleeve. I knew I didn't have to push myself. I didn't want to come back too quickly where it would hurt me long-term.

'I had to play with what I had for a few tournaments and that is why I didn't do any good. I would come in the middle or the back of the field at tournaments where the year before I had been finishing in the top five. It mostly pissed me off.'

It was a sign of how much desire Iles had, that he could make an astonishing recovery and still not be satisfied with his progress. He was miles ahead of where the doctors had thought he would be. He wasn't playing as well as the Bradley Iles of old, but he was still playing better than the majority of his elite peer group. It wasn't enough, though, for Iles. He felt that his instinct had been lost in the accident. Before, he had visualised each shot to the extent that he knew as he addressed the ball exactly where it would land. Now, he felt he was making it up as he went along. There were too many wild shots in his repertoire to put together a round that would cause his main rivals to take note. The junior champion had faded back into the pack and in the first few months of 2005, Iles began to doubt the realism of his dream.

'I always had hope and belief but there were times when I thought, "What if I'm never going to be able to understand this game again?" I always wanted to do something in golf but I was wondering whether I would ever be able to play it. It felt a bit fake. It didn't feel like I knew what I was going to do before I did it.'

Mediocrity didn't sit well with Iles. He could tolerate his reduced form up to a point. He hardly needed reminding of what he had been through. He was aware that he had come back way ahead of schedule so he could accept that it would take time before he was challenging for titles again. But this couldn't be him forever. He needed not only to be in the mix come the final round, but he also needed to start feeling more in tune with the game. As his father says: 'Prior to Brad's accident he would have been shooting five or six under the card and now he was shooting 14 over. He was quite disappointed that he had so far to go. That was a bit of a low point.'

Even when Iles finally got the sort of breakthrough he was after when he won New Zealand's North Island Amateur title in May, he still didn't feel any jubilation. He put his victory down to a combination of luck and the failings of his fellow competitors. He had won by default as far as he was concerned. His only option was to keep grinding away so he headed off to the States again as he had so fatefully done the year before. All he could do was keep playing and hope that in time it would all become second nature again.

The muscle memory that had been lost had to be reprogrammed. That recognition would allow Iles to self-analyse while out on the course and self-correct his swing. Repetition was the best way to do the re-programming. His brain needed to be forced into concentrating day after day, hour after hour. The more he played the better Iles would become. That didn't become entirely obvious while he was in the States. His scores continued to drop and his golf became more consistent. But, despite all the improvements, he still didn't feel like he was quite where he wanted to be.

That all changed, however, in November when he received an invitation to play at the Australian PGA. The invitation came after Michael Campbell, fresh from winning the US Open, suggested to the organisers they throw Iles a wild card. Campbell had been following the progress of Iles and believed the 22-year-old had something special to offer. It was a massive break for Iles. He had been slogging away since his comeback tournament in Hastings. In the early part of the year there had been plenty of rounds where the magic had deserted him entirely. He'd battled with his own physical limitations and suffered the frustration of not being able to play the way he felt he could. Struggling to make the cut in tournaments he had previously won seriously tested his resolve. But all the time he kept at it. He kept working on his swing with Mal Tongue. He kept going to the gym and he kept believing that, in time, he would make his mark as a professional golfer.

When he was invited to play at the Australian PGA he sensed that he had been given an opportunity that would have been criminal to waste, so he shot opening rounds of 71 and 69 to not only make the cut, but also to be challenging for the title.

His reward was to be drawn with Campbell and Australia's top golfer, Robert Allenby. The unthinkable had happened. From lying in a pool of his own blood only a couple of hours from death, Iles was walking with the giants. Campbell, Allenby and Iles – it had a ring that reverberated so pleasingly on the eardrums of the latter. The headaches, the nausea, the fatigue and the memory loss didn't seem so fresh in his mind now. He was living in the moment – and what a moment it was, not just for Bradley but for his father, too, who had vowed to caddy for his son in his first professional tournament.

'I was determined to go with him,' says Peter. 'When he was top of the leader-board I took a photo of it. That is one of the photos I will treasure for the rest of my life. He was ahead of Michael Campbell. It was amazing. I said to him when he was leading and we were walking down to one of his drives, "How are you feeling?" He said, "I'm feeling great." I said, "You look like a golfer," and he said, "Yeah, I feel like a golfer." It was all light-hearted. When he got paired with Campbell and Allenby that was such a big thing for him to hold it together with those two big names. He finished one over the card. He would have finished higher if he hadn't been paired with those guys but it prepared him for the next tournament.'

After shooting 73 in his third round, Iles closed out with a 71 to finish four under and tied for 26th place. He earned a cheque for $9552. He'd been tossed a golden ticket and he'd got maximum use out of it. But he didn't give two hoots about his payday. It was the fact he had played alongside some of the world's best players and hadn't looked out of place. It was then that he knew he belonged in such esteemed company. His accident hadn't stopped him fulfilling his destiny. It had maybe even enhanced his golf career.

When he arrived in Melbourne a week later to play in the Australian Masters at Huntingdale, he felt as if his whole life had been about preparing for that tournament. He shot an opening day 68, followed it up with a 69, struggled with everyone else on day three and carded a 74, before finishing in style with another 68. In only his second professional tournament, in a field that included seasoned professionals such as Craig Parry, Allenby and Stuart Appleby, Iles finished sixth.

'The turning point would have been the PGA – my first pro tournament. I realised I was back. That's when I knew I could play and that's a feeling I hadn't had for a year and a half. I knew then that I could play with these guys, if not better. The first three rounds of the PGA I was hoping not to make a fool of myself. After I stopped hoping I wouldn't go badly, I started saying, I can do this. I put on a different focus.

'It was amazing and then, at the Masters, it was even better. Before, when I was in the States, it felt like I was grinding. But at the Masters, it felt like I was born to be there.

'I wouldn't have got the invites to those tournaments if I hadn't had my injury. If people felt sorry for me I didn't care. I got the invite. If people see me as lucky getting these starts, so be it. But luck is a combination of preparation and opportunity. If you prepare well enough, when opportunities come along, you make the best of them. I played well.

'Mostly I think I am glad my accident happened. You just have to deal with it. That was the card I got dealt. I am in a lot better place now. I understand the world a lot better now. I live by the saying you are here for a good time not a long time. I know you are not guaranteed to be here for a long time.

'I want to be the US Masters champion. I want a green jacket. I don't really care if I'm not number one in the world or not the best golfer to come out of New Zealand. All I want is to win the Masters.'

There would be a cathartic irony should Iles ever succeed in winning the Masters. The tournament is played at the Augusta course in Georgia – not so very far from the scene of his accident. But presumably if Iles ever does win the Masters, he won't celebrate his triumph by heading out to look for alligators.

Bradley Iles holds cards to play as a professional on both the Australasian and Asian golf tours. He won his card for the Australasian Tour after his performances in the Australian PGA and Australian Masters in December 2005 and then came through a tough qualifying school a month later to earn his card for the Asian Tour. He is recognised as the most talented golfer of his generation by no less an authority than Michael Campbell. He has won several amateur titles in New Zealand, Australia and North America. Prior to concentrating on golf full-time, he studied Psychology at Victoria University in Wellington.

5

TAWERA NIKAU

New Zealand Kiwis 1990-1997 and
NRL Grand Final Winner 1999

Before 5 April 2001, the greatest tragedy in Tawera Nikau's life had been his infamous mullet. The tough Maori boy from Huntly had carved out a lucrative and successful rugby league career. He'd won a Grand Final with the Melbourne Storm in 1999, earned 19 test appearances for the Kiwis and was a legend at both the Castleford Tigers and Warrington Wolves. He was happily married and had two beautiful children. Apart from the hair, which by 1996 was committing heinous crimes against fashion, Nikau had only known success.

Then, on 5 April 2001, his world was torn apart. He'd come home from training with Warrington late in the afternoon as per usual. His wife, Letitia, wasn't so chipper, though. She told her husband she had been in town earlier that day and had copped some grief from the wife of one of the other Warrington players. The insinuation had been made that the Nikaus were in Warrington just for the money. Nikau had heard this kind of talk before. He'd been a professional league player for more than 10 years. He had learned to roll with the punches and accept that jealousy was a demon that some people struggled to contain. He wasn't dismissive of his wife, he just reminded her that they were too strong a unit to be knocked off their stride by gossip. A few more words were exchanged, just steam being blown off, and as Nikau flicked on the early evening news he was sure the whole issue had blown over.

But when Nikau headed to the garage a bit later – he had to pick up his son from his school play – he noticed the light was already on. And then he saw his wife, hanging. He scrambled for a hacksaw to cut her down, but it was too late. His attempts at mouth-to-mouth resuscitation were in vain. Letitia Nikau died on her way to hospital.

From standing on top of the world, Nikau was now tumbling into an abyss. The woman who had been the rock his league career was built on had inexplicably crumbled. There was no note. No suggestion something dramatic had been brewing. There was no history of depression, no episodes of sadness. The Nikau family home had only ever known the sound of laughter. Now it had to hear the eerie sound of grief. It was, and probably always will be, the hardest week of Nikau's life.

He was 34 and the love of his life, the woman he had met as a teenager in Huntly, had suddenly taken her own life. The heartbreak of losing someone so close was enormous. The fact that he couldn't understand why made it so much harder.

Then there were his children. Battling his own grief, he needed to be a strong father to them. He needed to help them through the most traumatic and harrowing time of their young lives. Heaven was 12 and Tyme was eight. They were not equipped to deal with such a tragedy. Somehow Nikau had to steer them through. He had to be their rock, the same way Letitia had been his.

'To lose somebody that meant everything and to overcome that … it's not easy,' says Nikau. 'The biggest thing was that we had two young children and my focus, I suppose, was on them. I channelled a lot of my energy into the children. It was one of those things that was really out of character for Letitia. She always planned things meticulously. She always had a Plan B. It didn't matter what we were doing, she always had it organised so it was really out of character for her to do this. There was no reason why.'

The grim reality of death prevented Nikau from immediately travelling down the torturous path of looking for answers. That would come. But first the practicalities had to be taken care of. Death doesn't just bring grief. It brings a bureaucratic burden. Those who have lost a loved one aren't afforded an immediate window to mourn. Instead, Nikau spent the week after his wife's death dealing with the paperwork. The police, the hospital, the morgue, they all needed to file reports and sign off official documentation.

By the time Nikau arrived back in Huntly with the body, he felt a massive weight lifted. His family had taken care of the funeral arrangements. He was back with his people, the whanau extended its loving arm and pulled Nikau and his two children tight into its fold.

'It was a big relief when I got back home. I knew that my family was there for me and that they would help me with all the funeral stuff. Going to the morgue, checking the body, having to do that on my own, that was the hardest part. But once I got home and had the support of my family and Letitia's family it was really good. Maori have a really good way of grieving. We do it for three days and really let it all out. Once it is over it is over. That is what the process is all about – getting that stuff out of you.

'Some people have breakdowns three or four years later because they didn't express their emotions at the time. Being brought up in the environment and going to funerals with aunties and uncles, that was our way and that was how I coped with it. I was pretty lucky that I had some good friends and family. It is what you are taught at a young age.'

There was so much to get out at the funeral, too. Richard Becht, a sports journalist for more than 30 years and the author of Nikau's biography, *Standing Tall*, can bring tears to his eyes by conjuring up specific parts of Nikau's testimony. Becht can remember interviewing Nikau in 2004. It was really the first time Nikau had talked about his wife's death to anyone outside his whanau or circle of friends. The big difference here was that this was going to be committed to print. His words and his emotions were going to be preserved for eternity.

'I can remember a line from the book that just about has me bawling every time I read it or think about it,' says Becht. 'When he told me the story of the day his wife committed suicide he said he and his two kids were sitting on the couch. Just holding each other and crying. It is an image I can envisage so clearly. The three of them, holding each other on this couch, in a house in a mining town in the North of England. It's very powerful.

'I think one of the things that has given Tawera his emotional strength is his spiritual understanding of his Maori culture. I could see that this was a man who had grieved plenty. That put him at ease.'

With the funeral out of the way and the emotion spent, Nikau had clarity. He knew that the right thing to do was to go back to Warrington and finish his contract. His whole career had been about giving of his best. He had always taken the view that he had to be professional in every facet. And maybe, more importantly, he felt it was what Letitia would have wanted him to do. Warrington had given him all the space he needed. If Nikau had called it quits there and then, they would have understood. But that wasn't his way.

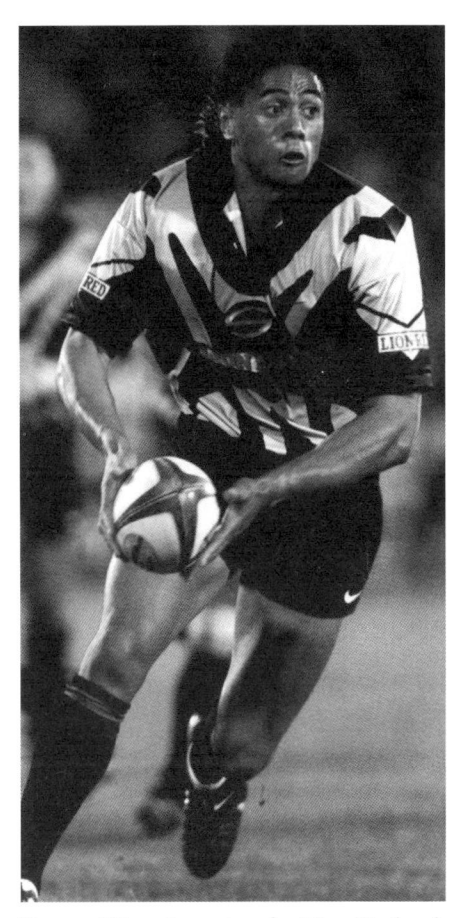

Tawera Nikau in action for New Zealand, 1997. *Glenn Jeffrey, New Zealand Herald*

'Letitia really would have wanted me to finish my contract. It was always important for me to be a professional. That is what we had been striving for and it was always our belief that if you were being paid to do something then that was your job. It was halfway through the season. She would have wanted me to get some closure in the UK.'

Once Nikau got back to the UK, he needed to adapt to his new circumstances. The kids had to be taken to and picked up from school. That was all right as he didn't normally start training until 10 am and was finished by 3 pm most days. There were friends willing to help out and it was always possible to get a babysitter so Nikau could squeeze in the odd night out. But coping with the practicalities was not really the hard bit, even though Nikau says: 'All I had to worry about with Letitia was playing football. She did everything for me.'

The emotional side of his life, understandably, was still in turmoil. He was trying to come to terms with the void. After 15 years together, that wasn't easy. Then there was the fact Letitia had given no reason why she had taken her own life. That proved a torture for Nikau.

He couldn't help but wonder whether he had said something or done something that had triggered his wife's actions. He didn't feel that he had. Nothing came to mind. The quarrel they had only hours before she died had been nothing. But he was still being torn apart by the agony of doubt. The guilt was overbearing. No matter how hard he tried, he couldn't stop wondering. It made him angry, bitter and frustrated. On the surface he could keep the emotions in check. Deep in the core, though, it was a different story. Maybe getting some answers would help him in his search for contentment.

But after a while he learned that he would never get any answers and he had to let it go. He was torturing himself by going down a road that had no start or finish, nor any directions. He learned to accept that Letitia had made a choice. It wasn't for him to judge whether it was right or wrong, he simply had to accept it. And as he came to terms with that, he began to ease away from the tragedy. It wasn't a case of forgetting, it was a case of storing the memories and carrying them in the proper place and using them to help move on with his life. He was still a young man. His life still needed to be lived.

Not surprisingly with so many contrasting and difficult emotions engulfing him, the passion for playing league dimmed as he saw out his career. He no longer burned with ambition and he went through the motions until the end of the season.

'Once I got back to England it wasn't too bad. It worked out pretty well. The main thing when you go through some adversity is it does change you. You have a philosophical view of life I suppose. You view things differently. I went through a period of differing emotions. A lot of the time I wondered what had happened. I was asking myself, why? I went through that for a period but I realised I couldn't carry on like that, otherwise I would end up going mad.

'I guess as a result of what happened I lost that fire in the belly. The reason I started playing was because I loved to play. Although I went back to finish off my contract, I had lost that spark. It was just about seeing out my time. I was holding up my end of the bargain and when I retired I knew that was the last game I would ever play. It was only about half a year. But it was pretty tough to get out there. It became a chore for me. I always said that when I got to the stage that I wasn't enjoying it I would retire.' And that's exactly what he did. He fulfilled his obligations with Warrington, then he came back to New Zealand to settle his kids in their homeland and to start building a coaching career and his business interests.

Being back with the whanau was important. The children had endured a turbulent experience and needed grounding. The anchor had to be put down. And where better than the family seat of Huntly?

The transition was smooth. League had only been a bit part of Nikau's life for the last few months so there was no sense of loss at no longer lacing the boots. If anything, it was a major relief to be freed of the grind of being obligated to a sport he no longer felt quite the same way about. Once back in New Zealand he was able to indulge himself a little. Buy those boys' toys he felt he deserved after almost 20 years of putting his body on the line.

And there was no bigger toy than the 1450 cc Harley Davidson 100th anniversary Fat Boy. That was his biggest indulgence. Motorbikes had been a passion since he could remember. Growing up on a farm, he had been riding them since he was big enough to reach the handlebars. But once he became serious about his professional league career, the bikes had to go. Strangely, league executives get a little nervy when they see

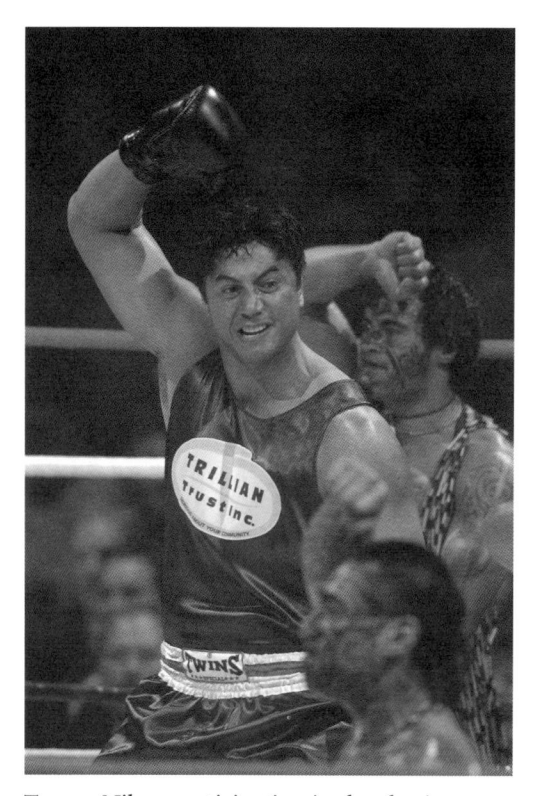

Tawera Nikau participating in the charity event Fight For Life in 2002. *Fiona Goodall, Suburban Newspapers*

their prize assets cruising at big speeds on two wheels. With no one to answer to any more, Nikau splashed out almost $45,000 on his Fat Boy. Well, the Fat Boy had to look good, so Nikau opted to have all the trimmings, including $6000 of mag wheels. It was those mag wheels that ended up causing a lot more bother than they were ever worth.

On 1 July 2003 Nikau took his Fat Boy into Hamilton to get the new wheels fitted. It was one of those glorious winter days, where if it hadn't been for the sun setting at 5 pm, there would have been little way of knowing it wasn't summer. He picked his bike up later in the day, by which time the Fat Boy was resplendent in its new garb. Nikau could barely contain his pride. He'd been knocked around muddy fields from Sydney to Brisbane, to London, to Huddersfield to Huntly. Seeing this wondrous concoction of chrome and rubber, well, it almost made it all worth it. The sun was shining, his children were doing well at school and readjusting to life in New Zealand and Nikau had a bike that all the other cool kids would have killed for.

And then it took just a second for 1 July to turn very sour. He was only a few minutes from home when his attention was distracted by some ducks taking off in the paddock next to the road. He came round the corner a little too near the centre line and was clipped by a Land Rover coming the other way. It wasn't major, but his leg got caught up in the

Land Rover's bull bars and as a result he was flipped into the air where he completed a half somersault, possibly with pike, and maybe even a twist. There was no grace about it, though. The judges would have scored it low and would have been particularly harsh on artistic merit.

By the time Nikau came to an undignified halt he was much like a James Bond martini — shaken but not stirred. His head seemed fine, his limbs were all accounted for and there was no obvious bleeding. Then he stood up and his right leg gave way. It was a broken leg. Nothing major. He thought it would be a couple of nights in hospital and then back home with a cast and enough embarrassment to fill a suitcase.

As he lay on the side of the road he called his brother to organise the kids and get his bike picked up. And then it was into the helicopter, delaying slightly to circle Taupiri Mountain so Nikau could pay his respects to his ancestors before heading off to Waikato Hospital.

He still wasn't unduly alarmed by his injury. That came a few days later when he was rushed to critical care to have his leg sliced open to release the pressure. His leg was infected and Nikau was no longer looking at a quick in and out job. He had to endure a series of operations over the next three weeks as the doctors tried to save the leg. His weight dropped from 130 kg to 80 kg. There was a tragic irony that his much-reduced form was going to be infinitely harder to mobilise. After three weeks of fruitless operating, the doctors were still only offering long odds on being able to save the leg. They narrowed the potential salvage options down to two.

The first was to stay in hospital for the next 15 months and subject himself to more operations. That might have worked, although, even if the leg were to survive, it would still only have limited mobility. The other option was to be done with it and have the thing lopped off.

For a man who had lost his wife in tragic circumstances just two years earlier, this was some way short of being a fair deal. But Nikau, as he had done when tragedy had invaded his life in 2001, thought not about himself, but about his children. Both Heaven and Tyme had been shocked to see their father so unwell. A clot in his lung had developed as a complication of the infection. He had already been in hospital for three weeks. The prospect of stretching that for at least another year was limited in appeal.

His children had endured enough. How would they cope if their father were removed from their daily lives? Nikau pretty much knew the answer to that and so it was, on 30 July, that he went into theatre to have his right leg amputated below the knee. When he came to, he was remarkably unfazed by his reduced limb. He was in a lot less pain and at last he could start thinking about getting home and getting on with his life. He had one little moment of self-pity.

'I wasn't angry or bitter about losing my leg. I did cry the day after I lost it and wondered what does a one-legged former rugby league player do? A big part of my makeup is my spiritual beliefs, not in the God sense but in the Maori context. That part of me has helped me overcome a lot of the issues I have had.

'Losing my wife and my leg within such a short time was pretty tough. But it is all about your attitude. The quality of life you will ultimately enjoy is not determined by what happens to you, but by what you decide to do about it. So the quality of my life was not going to be determined by losing my leg but by my attitude towards it and I have been a lot busier than I thought I would be.

'I am doing television work for Maori TV. I am coaching the Waikato side and doing some other TV stuff. When I went to hospital my brother's wife said something quite profound – she said, "Tawera's a good man but he will be a better man when he comes out of hospital."'

That it was just one moment of self-pity Nikau allowed himself is something that doesn't surprise his old friend, former Kiwi team-mate, Dean Lonergan.

'Tawera is, without doubt, the single most positive-minded person I have ever met,' says Lonergan. 'In all the time I have known him I don't think I have ever heard him say anything negative or feel sorry for himself. When he fell off his bike and lost his leg, he never once worried about himself. He was always thinking about his kids. If you need a favour Tawera will do it for you. He'd give you the shirt off his back if you asked. This all sounds pretty fawning, but there you go, I don't think anyone could have a bad word to say about the guy.'

Nikau used to have both legs and charge around with a football tucked under one arm. Now he has one leg and spends his time coaching and mentoring. There's a common thread that ties these two versions of the same man together – one leg or two, he's always been an inspiration.

Tawera Nikau played 19 tests for the New Zealand Kiwis rugby league team as well as playing for Castleford Tigers (1991–1996), Cronulla Sharks (1995–1997), Melbourne Storm (1998–1999) and Warrington Wolves (2000–2001). He helped Melbourne win the NRL Grand Final in 1999 and is still revered by the club. He is now an ambitious coach and astute judges say it won't be long before he is being considered for the biggest jobs. He has also made it a stated goal to compete at the Paralympic Games in track and field.

6

JUSTIN COLLINS

Northland, Chiefs, Blues and Auckland 1993–

When the hulking form of Kees Meeuws and his front-row chums chugged past, Justin Collins knew there was something wrong. Collins was a greyhound, Meeuws and his boys were St Bernards. There was no way Collins should be struggling to keep up. But he was. And that wasn't just an affront to his pride, it was a serious worry.

Collins led from the front at all of the Blues training sessions. It was a source of pride that his fitness levels were unrivalled in the squad. They had been since he was selected for the Blues in 1999. When he started pre-season training in 2002, he fully expected to once again be setting the benchmark for fitness. He didn't just expect it. In 2002 he demanded it, for there was a little extra incentive sizzling away in his tank.

A few months earlier he had been playing for Auckland against Otago in the NPC. Collins had, by his own admission, a stinker of a game. He'd struggled with the pace. Wherever the ball was he wasn't. He'd chased his shadow most of the night and returned to the dank changing rooms deep within the bowels of Carisbrook to brood over his own failings. He could sense that his body was unusually fatigued. His legs were uncharacteristically heavy and his lungs were heavy sponges, too bloated to suck in any air. Collins didn't ever get round to questioning his state of health that night. He got a far more blunt assessment of where he had gone wrong from the legendary Otago coach Gordon Hunter. Having coached Collins at the Blues in previous years their relationship was strong enough to survive a few home truths. 'Look boy,' opined Hunter in his none-too-frilly manner, 'you looked bad out there. You need to train harder.' Message received and understood, and so it was that come pre-season, Collins set off at a rattling clip in the first of ten 400-metre repeats the Blues would do that day.

It didn't take him long to feel like he had hit an iceberg of Titanic proportions. 'We were doing interval-training round the track. I'm usually a naturally fit person and top of the fitness levels for all the teams I have played in. I turned up to a session and I had a heart-rate monitor on. The first couple of intervals I led both of them. We were doing 10. By about number three I dropped back a bit and three or four guys overtook me. I wasn't feeling very good.

'Then by five and six I was coming last, front-row forwards included. I had all intentions of doing well. I would sprint out of the line like I normally would but I would just hit a wall. The whole pack would run past me. I could barely get one foot in front of the other. By the end I was coming last. Most of the guys had finished and I still had about 100 metres to go. The coaches came up to me and said, "Oh look, you pushed yourself a bit hard there and blew yourself out." But I looked at my heart-rate monitor and it was at 239 beats a minute and I was feeling awful. After another 15 minutes my heart-rate was still 180 beats a minute and that was after resting. I was trying to take my pulse but I couldn't count the beats. They were irregular, big, small and fast. So I thought there was something wrong.

'After that I made an appointment to see my doctor and he put me on to a specialist. He said there were a number of possibilities as there are many problems with the heart. He said he thought he knew what it sounded like but he needed to capture it on an ECG machine. He didn't really say too much about it. He said it would be some sort of fibrillation. The specialist has got a treadmill in his office so I ended up flogging myself for 15 minutes with a normal heart beat. So I had to wear a portable monitor to record

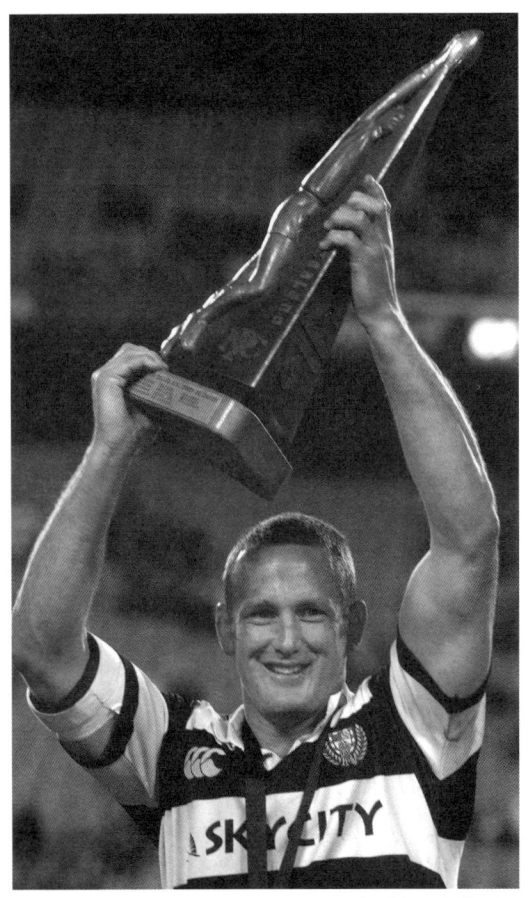

Auckland skipper Justin Collins holds aloft the NPC trophy at Eden Park, October 2005. *Suburban Newspapers*

it. When you feel your heart going out, and by that I mean when you feel this crazy, really fast, really irregular beating, you press the record button and you try and capture it.'

The big hope for Collins was that it was a one-off. He couldn't possibly get through a Super 12 campaign if his heart went into meltdown every time he put it under pressure. He was a loose forward. His engine needed to be finely tuned. But when he returned to training, he realised that the gods were not smiling. His heart, a previously staid and quite dependable piece of machinery, had somehow gone from Volkswagen to Skoda. At least once every couple of weeks it would suddenly start beating to its own wild and irregular rhythm. When that happened his legs turned to stone. His lungs would immediately start heaving and rugby became a labour every bit as tough as the tasks of Heracles. He was stuck in limbo, though, until he could capture data of his heart's peculiar samba. Without the facts, the diagnosis could not be made, and capturing the problem proved harder than living with it.

'I wore a portable monitor for a couple of weeks at training. I couldn't capture it but every now and then it would happen, my heart would go mad. I would only feel it maybe once every couple of weeks. I found that if I had a sudden burst of activity it would trigger the irregular beat. I can remember sitting watching TV, then suddenly running up the stairs at home and then feeling the heart going out and starting this irregular beat. I knew there was something wrong but the capturing of it was so hard.

'We were doing intervals again and I remember the heart went out so I said to the coach, "Look, I have got to go." I said, "I have got to go to the hospital and get my heart checked out." The team doctor knew about my problem. The coaches didn't know too much about it so I am not too sure what they were thinking at that point. I jumped in the car and raced to the hospital. What was happening was it would go out and when I stopped exercising it would go back to normal. They made me fill out a form when I got to the Mercy Hospital. I tried explaining that I really needed to get to the ECG machine as quickly as possible but they still made me fill out a form.

'I got in there after about 10 minutes and they laid me down. I had been running up and down the road outside while I was waiting, trying to keep the heart going badly. I whipped the shirt off and they tried to stick the electrodes on but I was sweating and nothing stuck and then my heart went back to normal.'

It was starting to become a major worry for Collins. These random episodes were becoming more frequent. He felt they were having a noticeable impact on his performance. There were times in a game when his heart would jump to its random beat and he struggled to get to where he needed to be. It was stretching him to the limit. He was playing one of the most physically demanding sports, in one of the most physically demanding positions for one of the world's premier provincial teams in the toughest provincial competition in the world and he had a serious but as yet undiagnosed heart condition. Understandably, it was playing on his mind, which in itself was another problem. The pace and intensity of Super 12 is such that you can't afford for the brain to have even a fraction of its focus anywhere other than the game.

Collins had acknowledgement there was a problem, but the exact nature of that problem couldn't be determined until there was better intelligence. And without knowing the exact nature of the problem, his specialist couldn't recommend any remedy. He had been sucked into a vicious cycle. It was a frustrating time for Collins and when the NPC came around that year, he was desperate for some sort of answer.

'It was starting to get worse, although I found if I got into it slowly and spent a long time warming up it wasn't too bad. If I got the heart-rate going up slowly then I tended to find I had fewer problems. But if something happened quickly it would trip out.

'I can remember being really fed up with the whole failure to capture it and then one day at Auckland training, my heart started beating really irregularly again. My heart was clearly not right, it was beating really fast with a strange rhythm, but I was sick of rushing to the hospital. I had dinner at Eden Park and it was still out so I drove past the hospital on the way home to see if it was still doing it. It was, and so finally, I got it recorded and then I went to see the specialist. He told me I had atrial fibrillation. There could be a flutter as well. He said there were a few things that we could try. There were a couple of different drugs. So after that meeting with the specialist I would take a couple of pills two hours before I would train or play. After taking those drugs, and if I warmed up slowly, I had no problems. By the end of 2002 I was feeling great. The problem had been diagnosed, the drugs were working and we won the NPC.'

After so long living with the unknown, Collins had his problem not only diagnosed, but well under control. There was even the added bonus of now knowing that his isolated horror performance in Dunedin had been due to his heart problem. When the Blues convened for their 2003 pre-season training, Collins would most definitely not be suffering the indignity of having the heavy brigade chug past him. His heart was beating as steadily as a grandfather clock.

The associated problems didn't kick in during that Super 12 campaign – a campaign won by the Blues and one many would say was Collins' finest. As the Blues blazed their trail to glory, Collins was at the core of everything they did. He was as fit as he had ever been and with the confidence that his heart was behaving, he could concentrate just on rugby. That was a luxury not afforded to him the previous year, as every few weeks he knew he would have to contend with an out-of-control heart and all the various fatigue-related issues that came with that.

If there was a downside to that campaign it was his failure to get recognised at the next level. He'd been selected to play for New Zealand A in 2000. Many astute rugby brains felt it would only be a matter of time before he made the jump to a full test cap. That time perhaps should have come in 2003 when he was, by most people's reckoning, the form blindside flanker in the tournament. However, acknowledgement from the only person that really mattered – All Black coach John Mitchell – just wouldn't come and he was left nursing that awful, close-but-no-cigar rejection professional athletes get no solace from.

A few months later, he'd have been delighted if his only problem was feeling a touch disappointed not to have made the All Blacks. When the 2003 NPC came around, as in the song by the Verve, the drugs didn't work. Collins was struggling. His heart was tripping out again. And it was tripping out more regularly and with greater severity. His capacity was reduced to about half.

'The drugs started not to work by mid-way through 2003. I would take the drugs before exercise but then the heart would trip out again. So I went back to the specialist. I was taking three different lots of drugs by then at different times of the day. I was getting quite down because I was trying my guts out. I was lucky I had a coach, Wayne Pivac, who was keen for me to play. But I knew I wasn't playing very well. I wasn't up to speed. I could only play one phase at a time. I would sprint out of a scrum and play that phase and then I would have to walk or jog slowly in between. I thought it was noticeable. I told Wayne that I would keep playing but that I didn't think I was playing very well. He knew all about it and he was happy for me to keep playing. I kept feeling I was letting people down. I felt like I looked like I was being lazy. We had won a couple of competitions and things were going well. But I thought people might think I was taking things for granted. I was getting down about that.

'Strangely, though, I don't think anyone did notice because we were playing well and we won the competition again. Some reporters would come up and say, "You must be really happy you are playing so well." I would say, "The team is going well." They helped me along. I couldn't start making excuses and say anything about it.'

It's easy to understand why Collins was concerned he was letting others down. He's known throughout football circles as a consummate professional. As someone who would rather die than let his mates or himself down. Aware that he wasn't able to perform to the level he felt was acceptable, Collins was paranoid he would be viewed as a phoney. When his pay cheque arrived every month, he wanted to feel that he had earned it. He might have been worried that he hadn't, but Pivac saw it all very differently.

'It's not that hard to manage Justin Collins even at the worst of times. He's the most professional player I have ever worked with. He's one of the hardest working and most honest professionals in the game and he was very upfront about his condition and how he was feeling. I would estimate that we were getting Justin at 75 per cent, but even at that level, he was still playing well enough to be selected.

'We weren't picking him just because he was Justin Collins. We were selecting him on form. There are a number of players who can buoy a team with their presence and he would be one of those players. When we reviewed his stats each week his tackle count was right up there, his arrival at the breakdown was right up there. He was still playing better than any of the other guys we could have picked.

'We were very aware of his problem but our advice from the medical team was that we would not be harming him by selecting him. He was taking his various drugs and as long as there was no long-term risk and he was playing well enough, we were going to select him. I guess some people might wonder why we didn't say anything public about Justin's heart, but he's just not the sort of person to make excuses. I'm sure he was also worried that it would have created too much media interest and put the focus on him and taken it away from the team.

'I think the best way to put things in perspective is to say that he'll go down as one of the unluckiest players not to make the All Blacks. If you look at his stats in 2003, they were consistently better than Reuben Thorne's, the incumbent All Black blindside. To outperform the All Black incumbent on stats alone with his heart condition, that says everything about how good he was.'

Collins, despite still being deemed good enough to earn his place in the Auckland team, wanted his problem fixed. When the drugs had been working during the 2003 Super 12, he had produced the form of his life. He couldn't go on having rest periods during the game. He needed to be able to compete at every phase and not have his heart dictate when he could get involved. He was close to 30. To win another Super 12 contract he would need to be at his best. How could the Blues, a franchise with more young talent than you could shake a stick at, contract a 29-year-old flanker with a dicky heart? Collins had to be able to give of his best to preserve his professional status.

His options were to try alternative drugs or to have an operation. Once given details of the operation he opted to push on with more drug therapy. The chances of the operation being a success were about 30 per cent. The chances of his condition staying the same after the operation were also about 30 per cent. The crazy figure that put him right off the idea was the 40 per cent chance of things being worse after going under the knife.

The other problem was that Collins would have to take a blood-thinning agent for eight weeks prior to the operation. That would prevent him playing as he wouldn't be able to risk being bruised while taking the drug. He desperately wanted to play in the 2004 Super 12 so the operation wasn't a valid option after the 2003 NPC. By the time he had taken the drugs for eight weeks and then rested after the operation, the Super 12 would have been and gone. He was contracted with the New Zealand Rugby Union until the end of 2004 so he felt he needed a big season to ensure he would be re-signing. It was decided, then, that Collins would use beta-blockers to help him through the last few games of the 2003 NPC.

At first he thought his luck was in. The drugs stopped his heart going into overdrive. His choice of solution, it seemed, had been the right one. But a couple of games after he started taking them, he knew there was no way the beta-blockers were going to get him through a competition as

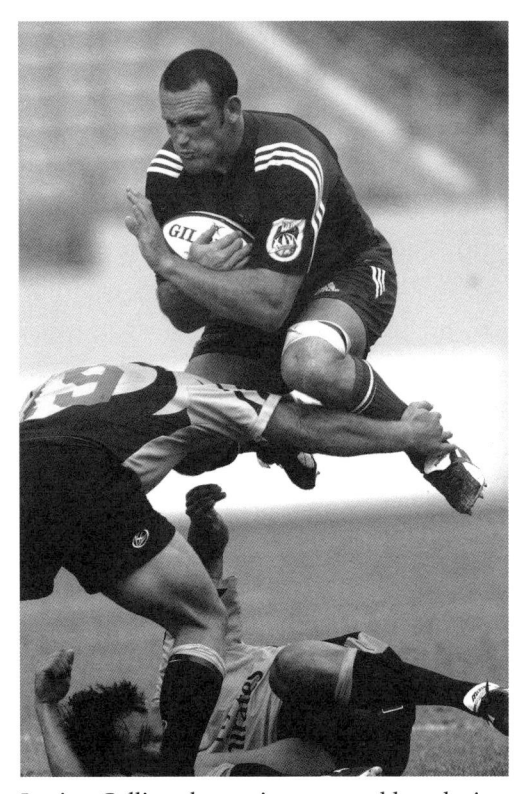

Justin Collins leaps into a tackle playing in a trial match for the Blues against the Western Force at Eden Park, February 2006.
Suburban Newspapers

physically demanding as the Super 12.

'We decided we would try beta-blockers. They slow the heart-rate right down. I was still taking all the drugs plus the beta-blockers and that seemed to work. I didn't have the irregular heartbeat. I could play again. What I found, though, was the beta-blockers were taking my resting heart-rate down to 35 beats a minute. I used to play in a heart-rate monitor. I would normally play at 165 to 180 beats a minute. With the beta-blockers I was playing at 125 beats a minute. My heart-rate couldn't get up and it couldn't cater for the blood flow and oxygen flow to the muscles. So I was fatigued again because the heart couldn't keep up with what I wanted to do.

'I was in the same boat. I couldn't perform again. I was just dragging myself through with the beta-blockers. It was pretty obvious they weren't working. The heart-rate was down, the performance was down. By pre-season 2004, I knew it was going to be an absolute struggle because I couldn't do it. I knew then I had to have the operation after the Super 12. I knew I had to play through and try to stick it out. I got through the Super 12 feeling terrible. The same things were popping up. We didn't do very well. Daniel Braid was injured and I had to play openside. Your fitness levels have got to be even more up there to wear number seven, but we had no options.

'I remember having to play openside in Brisbane. I was captain and I was shattered. The game in Brisbane compounded things because of the temperature. I wasn't comfortable. Again not many people knew about it. By the end of that Super 12 I was looking like I was old and slow and past it. These were the words that came out of Graham Henry's mouth after the Super 12. They were picking All Black trial teams then and I wasn't expecting to get a trial. But I bumped into him somewhere and he said, "You won't get a trial, you're looking a bit past it." He's always got a bit of a smile, but, excuse the pun, I took it to heart a bit. I knew I was looking past it so I was glad for his honesty. But I knew it was the heart so it didn't faze me too much.

'At that point I wanted to stand on the roof and say, "Look I'm trying my guts out but I can't do it." But I didn't want to make excuses for it. It was also a career thing. I had Super 12 selection coming up. I wanted to see if I could get it sorted before making some sort of public announcement. That ultimately could have affected my selection. So I wanted to get it sorted before too many people found out about it.

'By the end of the 2004 Super 12 I had exhausted all avenues so there was nothing left but the operation. I got on the Internet and I rang doctors because I wanted to find professional athletes who had had it done. I couldn't get any names. The operation was only six years old. I found out through a friend that former Taranaki player Andy Slater had it done. He retired because of his heart problem and he said, go and do it.

'I took the blood-thinning drugs and flew down to Christchurch. I wasn't that apprehensive. I had this will to keep playing rugby and this was the last option. As far as I was concerned this is what I had to do. They put me on the table and they go through a vein in your leg up to the heart. I was just slightly sedated and they went into the right ventricle and they made burn marks on the inside of the heart. Basically beats were being omitted inside the heart that weren't supposed to be there. To be general, a beat was being caught inside the heart. That's called a cardiac ablation.

'Then they go through the heart wall to do a pulmonary vein isolation and that can be quite dangerous going through the heart wall. But the surgeon said, "You are lucky. One in four people have got a hole through that chamber wall so we don't need to cut a hole." That was a stroke of luck I needed.

'The surgeon knew I wanted to go back and play professional rugby and he was quite happy to do the operation. I said, "How long before I can play?" He said, "Six weeks. No contact but you can start running in two weeks."'

The surgery had been smooth and he had the added bonus of a much shorter recovery than he expected. But Collins still didn't know whether the problem had been fixed. The only way to find out was to get back out and start running. This was his last chance. If the operation hadn't worked there would be no choice but to hang up his boots. He couldn't get through another campaign on beta-blockers. No way. He was in the Last Chance Saloon, needing a major stroke of luck to find his way to the door and directions to a less desperate place.

He returned to Auckland and a couple of weeks later he was doing some light training. It felt good. There were no problems. The heart just boom-boomed. There was no boom-bump-boom. Boosted with a little confidence after his early results, he began to build the training load.

'At the start of 2004 NPC I was doing light training and doing some running with the team. I didn't need to take any drugs. After the light training I started to build. I had a few problems but they said that would happen. That was hard. I had to remember that they said this would happen and just relax. Halfway through the NPC I was feeling good and doing contact training. I ended up playing a couple of games for Auckland B and then for Auckland, coming off the bench against Southland.

'I wanted to show I was a success and I wanted to play Super 12. Blues coach Peter Sloane watched me in a handful of games after my heart surgery and asked how I was feeling. I said "Great" and he said, "I'm happy with that."'

And with his selection in the Blues 2005 squad and a two-year contract signed with the New Zealand Rugby Union, Collins could at last make some sense of the last few years. All those games he played where he could barely lift his leaden legs could be confined to a dark recess in his mind. His problem had been fixed, permanently.

There was also the added relief of having gone public with his heart condition. Once he knew the operation had been a success and that he would still be able to play professionally, Collins opened that particular window to the press. He was free, at last, to give all he had on a football field. All he had wanted for the last 24 months was the opportunity to finish his career with dignity and respect intact.

Maybe people who had watched him play in that period had seen no deterioration in his performance. To the rugby public his form had maybe dipped from the heights of that 2003 Super 12 campaign, but no one had noticed a collapse. That didn't matter to Collins, though. What mattered was that he felt he hadn't given of his best and the opportunity to rectify that was enormous. It is also an opportunity he has most definitely taken. He was made captain of Auckland for the 2005 NPC and led his side through a stunning revival. In 2004 Auckland were being labelled a disgrace. In 2005, with Collins guiding them, Auckland made it to the final where they easily beat Otago to be crowned NPC champions. The skipper gave them an edge they were so sadly missing when he was absent.

'It makes me pretty proud because of the way things could have gone. To be captain of Auckland, it has turned out pretty well. I don't need to tell anyone now. If anyone who did look at me and think he is off, they now have the reason. It wasn't because I was old and lazy. I'm glad the way it turned out.

'If the operation hadn't worked I was resigned to the fact I would only be able to play club footy. I was struggling so much before that I knew that if it didn't work it was over. All the doctors, all the trainers and all the coaches knew about my condition before I went public. And my closest friends Steve Devine and Xavier Rush knew about it. There were maybe only a handful of others who had been around enough to see me turn up to train with funny monitors on who also knew about it. That made it really hard for me within the team. I was feeling I didn't want to let my mates down when I was supposed to be somewhere to make a tackle.

That is why I made it clear to the coaches about how I was feeling. I just wanted things open and most of the time they wanted to pick me. Some of the players may have looked sideways. I don't know.

'The heart thing did hold me back. There could have been opportunities. I feel like it has been a pretty hard road. There have been some bloody good players that I have been competing with. I have given it everything. I tried and I wasn't good enough for whatever reason to make the All Blacks. It just wasn't my time. I don't let it worry me. I'm still playing professional football and it could have been a lot worse than that.'

It could have been so much worse. He could have bowed out as that bloke who used to be quite good. He could have left the game having threatened to make a footprint only to leave with little trace. But that will not happen. Justin Collins has made an indelible mark on New Zealand rugby. Brave and inspiring to the end, he doesn't need a black shirt to convince anyone he is a legend.

Justin Collins first played for Northland as an 18-year-old and went on to represent the province 75 times. He made the Chiefs Super 12 team in 1998 before shifting to the Blues, for whom he played in 2006 – his eighth consecutive season – before rupturing his Achilles in the second round. He was considered a key player in the Blues championship-winning team of 2003 and deemed unlucky by many astute judges not to have made the All Blacks that year. He transferred to Auckland in 2000, helping them to NPC titles in 2002, 2003 and as captain in 2005. He is contracted with Auckland until the end of 2007. He is married to Justine and has two daughters.

7

PETER TAYLOR

*Assistant Manager Canadian Equestrian Team
Barcelona Olympics, 1992*

There have been some legendary tales of sacrifice made by elite sportspeople. It would come as a surprise, however, to find any athlete who could trump Peter Taylor in terms of what he was prepared to do to make it to the Olympics. So strong was his desire to conquer equestrian sport, he thought nothing of becoming a prostitute to fund his passion.

For Taylor, prostitution was just another extraordinary chapter in a quite extraordinary life. He had been resourceful since the age of eight. That was the time he became the man of the house. He was absurdly young to be the domestic boss, but with dysfunctional parents, that was his lot. Growing up in the affluent Whangarei suburb of Kamo, Taylor's life should have been idyllic. It should have been about long, sun-drenched summers and happy times. But it wasn't. His was a lonely and tortured existence.

Aware that he was different and riddled with stress from his unhappy home life, little eight-year-old Peter Taylor started to become not so little. He started to find comfort in food and Peter Taylor became Tubby Taylor, everyone's favourite fat little odd-ball to pick on. That life could be cruel was a lesson Taylor was learning at an alarmingly young age. But, in a display of the resilience that was to be at the forefront for much of the rest of his life, Taylor adapted to his environment. The bullying hurt. The troubles at home upset him. But they also taught him one of the most valuable life lessons – that he couldn't trust anyone and if he wanted to instigate change, he would have to do it himself.

While that particular acorn was being planted in his brain, so was another that would also blossom into a significant oak tree in his life. Having been rejected and hurt by so many humans, Taylor found it hard to love. Until, that is, he discovered horses. Horses were capable of unconditional love. Horses didn't call you names or let you down. They were, in the eyes of the teenage Taylor, the most wonderful beasts to roam the earth. He had found true love.

'When I was eight I ran our house. I did the cooking and organised my two sisters. At that time life became a reality for me. I knew then that I had lost trust in my parents. I knew I couldn't trust anyone. For me to have any way of doing anything different in my life, I had to believe in myself. That may sound profound, but it was a simple process of survival.

'I started putting on weight and I was a bit of a loner. I guess there were a couple of things – I knew I was different but I didn't know why. I turned out to be gay but I just thought then I was a bit more sensitive. I wasn't very blokey. I was much more responsible. I was a golden retriever rather than a Jack Russell. My mother was a midwife and worked mainly on night duty. At school I was being bullied for being the fat kid. But I was also appreciated for being the most responsible. So although I was never picked for the team – nobody wanted Tubby Taylor – there was always that loveable nature to me. I would come in last on the cross-country run and everyone would clap. So there was a sense of acceptance.

'Because of the family experience, bullying became a watershed for me. I didn't buy into it. I couldn't beat them up. I couldn't run away so I ignored it. I appeared on the outside not to be hurt by it. I had a friend at school who was a redhead. He was the other boy who was always last to be picked for every team. He had a pony. We became good friends. I found it very difficult to love anybody so I directed my love to a horse. This became a way for me to show my passion and my genuine ability to love.'

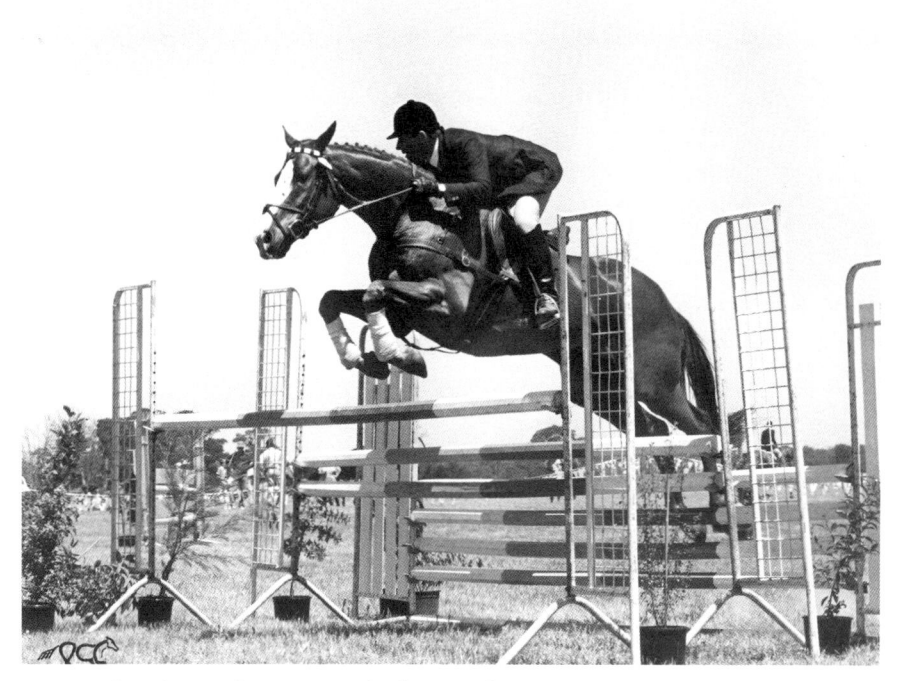

Peter Taylor clears a fence on Look Sharp at the 1988 Bi-centennial three-day event in Hawkesbury, New South Wales.

But that love was put on hold when he left school and decided to take off to Australia in search of smoother waters and adventure. He needed to get away from New Zealand and see the world. He had been working as a hospital orderly and he and a co-worker fled to the bright lights of Sydney. The problem was the co-worker thought they were more than friends. When he discovered the love would go unrequited, his suicidal tendencies bubbled to the surface. Racked with guilt and fearful he had led his friend on, Taylor gave him nearly all his money so he could fly back to New Zealand.

That left Taylor with 20 cents and a suitcase full of clothes in a railway station locker. He was still only 17. It was going to require a very neat trick or a very kind bounce to get him out of his predicament. He kind of got both.

'I thought I would catch my thoughts as I sat in some bar on Pitt Street. I bought an 18 cents glass of beer, which meant I no longer had any money. A guy started chatting to me. I assumed he wanted to have sex, which was quite the norm. But he didn't. He was heterosexual. He offered me his couch for the night. He offered to drive me back into town in the morning and on the way he started telling me about himself. He was the manager of Buckingham Men's Wear store and he said he needed to find a salesman for his store. He said, "Can you sell?" I had never sold in my life, but I knew I would be able to do it, so of course I said I could. The job was mine and he dropped me off at the railway station so I could pick up my suit. I started at 8.30. I learned very quickly how to measure people.

'When it came around to lunchtime, I was hungry and it was then that I realised I had no money. I went outside the store to have a think about what I could do and as I did, a bus went past with an advert for Lifeline and it said, "If you need help call this number." So I memorised the number and went back to the shop and called it. I told the person who answered the phone that I needed somewhere to stay and that I would be able to pay as I had a job.

'She gave me the address of a place where breakfast was included for $9 a week. Being an entrepreneur, I said I would organise breakfast for everyone in return for free rent. They said that was fine. So I got up 15 minutes earlier and prepared everyone's breakfast and tidied up. I had them trained in two days and I had free rent. What sounded like a tough time as a kid turned out to give me an enormous range of skills. I was clever and streetwise. I knew how to move around people. I knew how to charm people and tell them what they wanted to hear.'

He certainly knew what to tell the administrators at the Sydney catering college he applied to shortly after. Taylor had left school with no formal qualifications. He perhaps didn't give that impression on the application. Three years later, when he returned to Auckland to set up Le Brie restaurant with two friends, that hardly mattered.

And by then he was too busy to care if there was a white lie rattling around in his subconscious. His life had become all about the restaurant, working horrendous hours under intense pressure. All work and no play made Peter a dull boy. He needed an outlet and that's when it hit him. Horses, in all their equine glory, were missing from his life. His Australian adventures had not afforded him the time or finance to indulge in his favourite sport. But back in Auckland, where there was a wad of cash starting to burn a hole in his pocket, he could rekindle that passion for riding. And he needed to, even if it was just to get him out of the restaurant on occasion.

'I eventually graduated from college in 1975 and opened Le Brie restaurant in Auckland. I was head chef. After about 18 months I had lost weight, I had a successful business. So I wanted to take up riding again as a hobby on a Sunday. I was working six days a week.

'I bought a good horse and I started competing. There was a club in the evenings not far from where my horse was. There was an international trainer of great repute called Karl de Jurnack whose second wife lived on the North Shore. He would teach on a Thursday night and we all paid him in kind. I brought him food from the restaurant. By this time I had an amazing horse called Nirvana. I remember one night Karl said to me that he thought I had talent and that I should train. I said I didn't have time with the restaurant.'

But the encouragement of de Jurnack lit a fire within Taylor. Being praised was not something he expected. Nor was it something he had experienced much and it made him realise for the first time that there could be an avenue worth exploring. That was Taylor's way. He believed in succumbing to his passions. He wasn't the type to keep them underground and only let them out for a run when the late night booze kicked in. No, he wasn't the type to die wondering or bore his audience with empty talk. He was going to chase his dreams. The restaurant had become too big a part of his life. He was preparing entrees when the only place he wanted to be was on the back of his horse. He knew he couldn't let the chance pass him by, so he took a six-month break from Le Brie.

That break was spent at the National Equestrian Centre, learning under the legendary Lockie Richards. It was there that Taylor learned the foundation skills of his sport that would enable him to travel the world in his quest for Olympic glory.

When his six months were up, he didn't want to head back to Auckland and the life of a head chef. He was on a mission to make it to the summit of the equestrian world and he would do whatever it took to get there. That meant leaving New Zealand to compete on the European circuits. That was where he could hone his craft and compete with the best. He had a thirst to learn and working as a contract rider, topping his income with jobs in the hospitality sector, was the way to go.

But no sooner had he made up his mind and taken the plunge, than disaster struck.

Competing in his first international event in Belgium, his horse, Fez, was pricked by a blacksmith when being fitted with a new shoe. Taylor and Fez competed, oblivious to the fact that the horse had developed an infection called osteomyelitis. Less than five weeks later Fez was dead. Taylor's Olympic dream was virtually over before he'd even unpacked. It was a massive setback. Fez was a genuine Olympic-standard horse. Finding a replacement would be neither easy nor cheap. Taylor, though, was no stranger to adversity and had never before given up at the first sign of trouble. He knew from his time as a bullied child that perseverance would deliver results. And he knew from his adventures in Sydney that good fortune could be lurking round the next corner.

And so it was. A German trainer had seen him ride in Belgium and Fez or no Fez, she wanted Taylor to come to her stables and keep learning his sport. When he agreed, he effectively signed himself to a life of international equestrian competitions during the summer, punctuated with casual work wherever he could find it in the winter. That was his life, more or less, for the next decade. It was lived in that vein for the simple reason that Taylor wanted to give himself the best chance of making it to the Olympics.

The story of Taylor is a story of sacrifice. As he competed in Europe and North America, he was never the star rider. He was competent rather than spectacular. The big break just wouldn't come. He couldn't convince selectors he was in that top tier of a sport in which New Zealand was ruling the world at that time.

But the sub-plot of Taylor's life in many ways makes more fascinating reading. Owning and maintaining a world-class horse is not cheap. Operating as a contract rider gave Taylor a major problem, as contract riders were not in the big league of remuneration. Then there was the additional problem that horses take years to become world class. It's a delicate business training young horses from geldings to world champions. With the Olympics coming every four years, the timing can be tricky. Horses need to be at their peak at the right time and few competitors have the luxury of being able to run a stable so that they might get lucky with at least one of their options. It's a case of having one horse on the books and hoping it can make it to an Olympics in its prime.

Taylor was prepared to do anything to find the money he needed. He could have given up a thousand times. He could have accepted that only those fortunate enough to have been born into the right bank accounts can succeed in equestrian sport. He never did, though. He never saw the obstacles in his way as insurmountable.

Which is why, when he felt he had exhausted every avenue in his efforts to get to the Olympics, he was prepared to give prostitution a try. 'Usually, if I was working at a stable, I would also work in a bar at night. I was always able to use hospitality to supplement my income. When I got to London I had a job as a waiter but I also went for a job as a massage therapist. I thought I had handled enough bodies so that would do me. It was at the Burlington Men's Health Club in Old Bond Street. The men took off their bowler hats and we would take their shoes so they couldn't leave without paying. It was £22 a time. They said I was too old but they asked if I could be the receptionist.

'One of the clients came in and asked for me. He said he didn't want a therapist, that he wanted me. I told him I didn't finish work until 4.30. He asked me to meet him and I said, "It will cost you £50." I had a fantastic time and stood at the train station with £50 in my hand and thought that was the best hour's work I had ever done. It was so empowering. I was completely in charge of the whole situation.

'A few years later I was in Australia and I wanted a new horse and I needed money. I was running a restaurant on the Gold Coast, cooking omelettes. I was on the nudist beaches during the day playing backgammon for money. I was working for $3.50 an hour and I asked for a raise to $5. They said I was a tourist and I got $3.50 or nothing. I was

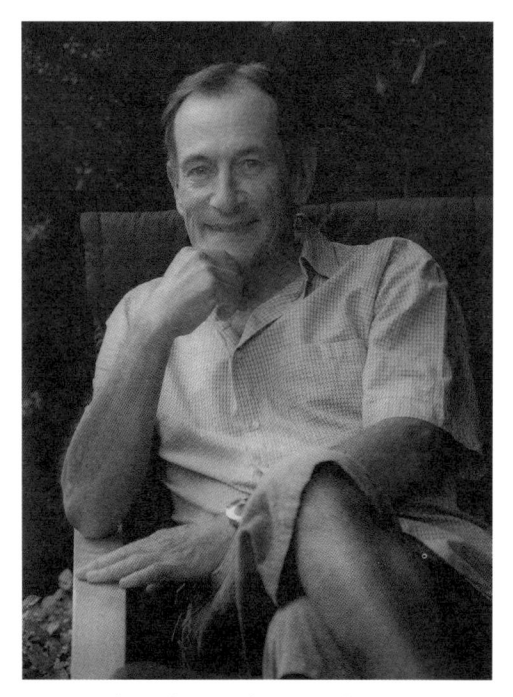

Peter Taylor relaxes at home today.

fired. So I went to Sydney to be a hooker.

'Not for one second did I have any issues. I was in charge. I decided whether it was yes or no. It was a way of making money. I went in empowered. I didn't even do an interview because I made it sound like I was an experienced hooker from London with my one client. But I knew the lingo from working on reception. I was being a genuine escort. I was there to raise money to buy a horse to go to the Olympic Games.'

But by 1990, Peter Taylor realised that his dream would be unfulfilled. There is no question he gave things his best shot. His sacrifice had been massive. He'd contracted HIV in the late 1980s. It was a setback, just like all the others, that he took in his stride.

Physically he was fine, although the threat of contracting AIDS was never far away. He was never going to make any allowances for his condition. The only major hindrance came in 1988 when, after competing in five three-day events in Australia, Taylor discovered his T-cells – a type of white blood cell crucial to the immune system – were dangerously low. He had to endure an eight-week drug trial. That was it. That was the only time he pandered to HIV.

Having devoted so much emotion, time and financial resource to his Olympic dream, it was with heavy heart that he decided to jack it all in and head back to New Zealand. Many on the equestrian circuit were puzzled as to why he was giving up when they thought he was so close. But Taylor had no money left to fund his passion. He just didn't have the fight left in him to put himself through another two gruelling years with only an outside hope of making it to Barcelona.

Back in New Zealand, he gave his horse to a trainer called Nicoli Fife to look after. From there the horse, Look Sharp, ended up being bought by top Canadian rider Nick Holmes-Smith. And bizarrely, just when it seemed Taylor had finally given up on his Olympic dream, it all happened for him. Taylor had gone to Pukekohe to watch Look Sharp at an event. As he was leaving he saw the horse tied to the back of a trailer with no water, rug or human company. Taylor vented his feelings on Holmes-Smith. The upshot was that Taylor left Pukekohe as Look Sharp's manager.

The relationship blossomed and when the Canadian team qualified for the 1992 Olympics, Taylor had worked his way into the position of assistant manager. Cinderella was at last going to go to the ball. Taylor arrived in Barcelona through the most circuitous route. His adventures were improbable, his sacrifice unparalleled. He most certainly didn't fit the norm in terms of profile and background. But what he had done to get there, what sacrifices he had made, what he had been prepared to do to fund his ambition – that was no one's business but his own. It didn't matter. All he had ever cared about was making it to the Olympics.

'I ended up at the Olympic Games but not as a rider as I originally hoped. I was there for the Canadians as their assistant team manager. There was a slight sadness that I didn't make it as a rider. But there was also an immediate recognition that I didn't quite have the talent. But when I got to the international level, working as a coach and as a trainer, I knew then that I could have done it as a rider. It wasn't that hard. If it had been my original horse I would have been there.

'Some of the other people on the team knew my story. Very few of them knew I had been a hooker. It wasn't of consequence to anyone else. I have learnt that people are very quick to judge. I was the only out gay man on the North American equestrian circuit. It wasn't important to me that anyone should know. I have always been task-orientated. That means it didn't matter how I got there. All that mattered was that I was there. I was respected for my job and I was highly efficient. I was also a lot of fun.'

There was, however, one cruel, ironic twist of fate to be endured. Having spent the better part of his adult life chasing a place at the Olympics, Taylor may have wished he had never succeeded. In April 1996 he suddenly felt dramatically unwell. He was confined to bed after contracting a bad fever and extreme dizziness. Tests were run and without being able to find anything specific, it was assumed he was suffering from a rapid progression of his HIV. By October he was deteriorating and his spleen had grown almost to the size of a football. He was told, best-case scenario, he had eight weeks to live. And true enough, when eight weeks had elapsed he was slipping out of this world.

He was in a coma a few days before Christmas but just as he seemed to be checking out, he eased his way back into life. The reprieve had been granted and no one knew exactly why. Until February 1997. That was when, after some serious detective work by his doctor, he was asked if he had ever been bitten by a sandfly. The answer was yes. Sandflies had been rife at the Barcelona Olympics and he remembered being ravaged by the blighters while spending most of his time in the stables. He was diagnosed with visceral *Leishmaniasis donovani* – a microscopic parasite that lives on dogs and rodents. The parasite attacks the internal organs, causes fever, anaemia, weight loss and an enlarged spleen.

The fact Taylor is still alive today says everything about his ability to conquer the impossible. He is smashed every few weeks with massive doses of chemotherapy and takes around 250 pills every week. He is now mostly blind. Yet, his spirit has not been crushed and he continues to defy medical science. No one else with both *Leishmaniasis* and HIV has managed more than 20 months. Taylor has managed eight years. He knows why.

'One of the interesting things about overcoming an illness is that if you have already had years of training to be disciplined, to be thinking positively, to be goal-setting, to be extraordinarily hard, it is a continuation of your life. I have had a life generated over years and years to direct me in a way that means I have to be mentally and emotionally strong. No one else in the world has lived longer with this illness; somehow I am the only one who keeps living. I am so far out of the outliving box I stopped being an international case study because everyone else was dying after two or three months. Now I have gone back to being a case study because I'm still living and my body keeps adapting to the environment it is in.

'I put this down to years and years as an athlete. That is to be well-informed, to be a great listener, to have a work ethic, positive attitude, and to be physically and mentally strong. Then, when it came to my health, it seemed to be not such a great challenge.

'I had to ask how was I going to keep going with this illness that was supposed to have killed me? I have outlived all the indicators. I am in a box of one. My state of mind is always at the forefront. When I say there is a window of opportunity that means I always look forward. I don't let it own me. I co-exist with it. Because I am available for opportunity, I never let one slip through my fingers. The whole premise to me is that I always focus away from myself. I am always pushing away from my comfort zone. Psychologically that is very important. You can either take four minutes to get over something or the rest of your life.

'I think I have had an enormous privilege. You need a lot of different tools to get through different situations in life. I am fortunate because so many things have been chucked in my toolbox.'

There will probably, in the world of equestrian sport at least, never be another toolbox quite like it.

Peter Taylor enjoyed an international equestrian career that saw him compete at the highest level for the better part of two decades. The highlight of his career was travelling to the Barcelona Olympics as an assistant manager to the Canadian equestrian team. He also enjoyed a rewarding business career as one of the founders of Le Brie restaurant in Auckland and later opened one of Auckland's first gay bars – Surrender Dorothy. He has lived the last 10 years of his life with the rare disease Leishmaniasis donovani.

8

TIM LYTHE

Auckland Aces Cricketer 2005–

The summer of 1999 arrived with heightened expectation for Tim Lythe. It would bring with it the welcome sound of leather crashing into willow. Soon, all the green spaces round Auckland would be echoing with cries of 'Howzat'. And for Lythe, a hugely promising 19-year-old off-spinner, the summer of 1999 would hopefully also bring his coveted first cap for Auckland. It would be a summer of fulfilled dreams – of that, Lythe was certain.

It was late October and Lythe had just returned from the UK, where he had been practising his craft for a club side in Bristol. He'd spent six largely idyllic months tweaking his off-breaks in the shadows of church spires on village greens across Gloucestershire. The theme of his trip was self-improvement. There was an acknowledgement that travel would broaden the mind. But really, Lythe was hoping the biggest improvements would come on the cricket field. His passion for cricket knew no bounds. It was almost as if the pop group 10cc had written their best-selling song *Dreadlock Holiday* with Lythe in mind, for indeed it was true: he didn't like cricket, oh no, he loved it.

Lythe came from a sports-mad family and cricket had been locked into his heart from the moment he could turn his arm over. As a pupil at

Mount Albert Grammar School Lythe turned his hand to many sports. It was always cricket, though, that captured his imagination. The heritage, the tactics, the nuances of spin bowling – he just loved the intricacies of the game. It helped no end that he was rather good at it. Good enough to be selected for the Auckland Under-19 team, and at the end of his last season in the age-grade side, the full Auckland team picked him as 12th man. He'd been close enough to smell the linseed oil being rubbed on the pros' bats. But he wanted more than a sniff. Lythe desperately wanted to be out in the middle, taking wickets and smashing a few to the boundary.

When the chance came up to spend a few off-season months in the UK, he jumped. While his compatriots would be confined to indoor net sessions during the New Zealand winter, he'd be honing his skills by playing in competitive matches. His was a difficult art. He could learn an enormous amount about flight and spin in the very different atmospheric conditions in the UK. The standard was only so-so, but he added some vital experience to his armoury.

When he got back to New Zealand there were just a few more tricks up his sleeve – a little bit of extra knowledge in the bank. He'd also refined his batting strokes. So it was no wonder that when he touched down in Auckland after his UK sojourn, he was desperate to get his right arm immediately back into action. He just needed to get a minor problem on the back of his knee sorted out and then he would be into it. It really was minor. His left leg felt a bit tight, that was all, and he could feel a small lump. His sister, a qualified physiotherapist, recommended a sports doctor and Lythe was sure that he would pop along to the surgery and the problem would be identified as either a cyst or a bone spur. He was facing only a couple of weeks, maximum, on the sidelines. His world caved in when he heard that the lump was in fact a cancerous tumour.

'I had felt a lump, about the size of a golf ball, when I was in the UK but never thought too much of it,' says Lythe, seven years on. 'The lump wasn't painful as such. It was more restrictive in terms of movement. The thought never crossed my mind that it was a tumour. I had really developed as a player and as a person while I was in England and I wanted to have everything right and crack into the season. I had a feeling I was on the verge and wanted to see what I could do. There was all this big excitement and then to have it taken away like that was devastating.

'I remember when they told me I had cancer, my first thought was that I would never play cricket again, not that there might be some consequences for my life. It is strange when I look back on it now, but that is how engrossed I was in sport.

'I had some X-rays and the sports doctor basically knew what it was and he referred me on to an orthopaedic surgeon. I wasn't sure what the first doctor was talking about at that stage. He was using the word osteosarcoma. It was the specialist who told me I had cancer. It blew me away that my life was in danger and that I would never play cricket again. Sport was my whole identity and my life revolved around cricket.'

Lythe felt like he had been hit for a very long six. His head was reeling. It took just seconds for his dreams to be stolen and then burned in front of his eyes. There would be no appearance for Auckland in the 1999-2000 season. There would be no appearance for Auckland the season after that. And here was the hammer blow – there would be no appearance for Auckland, period. He needed, though, to set aside that calamity and ensure that he avoided the far bigger one that had heaved into view.

He had a rare strain of bone cancer. It caught the medics on the hop. They were uncertain as to exactly what they were dealing with. Quite soon after the initial diagnosis they took a biopsy. There were theories as to the true nature of the cancer but they wanted to play safe and get advice from some experts in the United States. It would take a few weeks to get the results back. They would be agonising weeks for Lythe.

'I guess when they sent the biopsy off I stepped back and realised that cricket was not the major drama. I can remember there were times, particularly waiting for the results when I thought, this is really scary. They could tell you that you are stuffed. And then it would be bugger sport. That's when you get the shits. Waiting for those results I was beside myself. I never really thought about it until the day before, until it was right there. Maybe it was a human response to shut it out and pretend it was not there. That was how I treated a lot of my treatment and recovery – I almost had the view that it wasn't happening.

'People said I was so positive, but it was more that I didn't want to deal with it. Then there would be moments when reality would actually hit and I would think that there might be bad news tomorrow. That's when the fear and worry is immense. It was the worst thing. There was no answer. So I shut it out. I struggle to remember a lot of what happened. I read Lance Armstrong's book after my treatment and that was good because when I read about what happened to him it struck a chord with me. The way he described things reminded me of what I went through and sort of pieced it all together. The treatment and the feelings that he wrote about, I thought that was right.

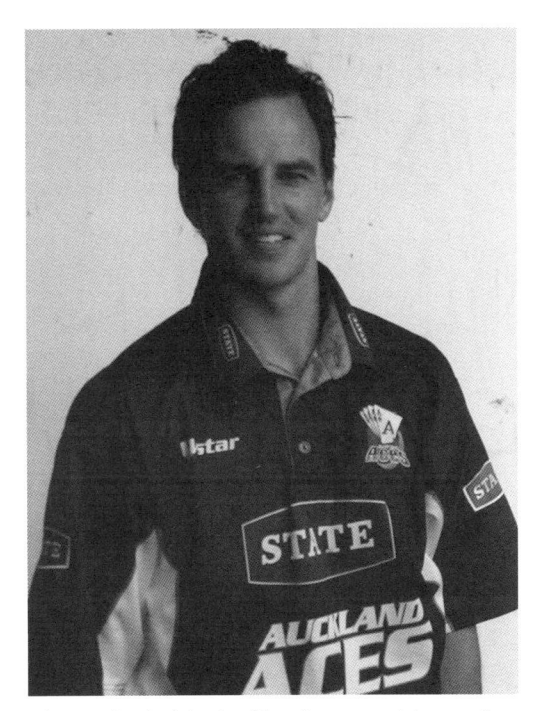

Tim Lythe in his Auckland gear waiting to bat against Wellington at Eden Park, January 2006.

'When the biopsy came back, they didn't really know how severe my cancer was. They weren't sure how bad it was so they treated it as if it was high grade. In early 2000 I started chemotherapy. I had three rounds and then I had surgery to cut out the tumour on the back of my femur right down to my knee. They cut quite a wide margin. They took half the femur out, all of the knee and ligaments. They replaced it with a metal rod and a plastic hinge joint. They took a large margin to ensure they got it all. There was some uncertainty as to how far the cancer had gone.

'I had some more chemotherapy in late 2000. They still gave me chemo to make sure it didn't spread. They always said they would do six rounds of chemo. It was brutal and I wouldn't wish it on anyone. They wanted to prevent any secondary sites. They never really knew how it would work but the treatment was successful. I think chemo is a bit like that. It is a bit hit and miss.

'At the end of the day it is luck. I was lucky enough to get it caught early before it had spread. There is no magic formula. It might have helped that I had a positive attitude, but I was just lucky. I think about what if someone wasn't a sportsperson and as active as me. They would never have noticed. Before they would have known it would have been too late. After my treatment was finished they said I would never jump or run.'

It didn't really require years of medical training to make the statement that Lythe would never jump or run again. It was obvious to anyone who caught sight of the withered limb that it was not going to be capable of much more than the most basic support role.

His prosthetic knee was a smart bit of kit. If he had fallen ill 30 years ago, Lythe would most probably have had his leg amputated, while even just five years ago he would have had only a crude device fitted, although amputation would have been a very real possibility then too if it was found that the cancer had spread beyond the site of the surgery. So he was reasonably fortunate that as a man of the new millennium, he would have a level of mobility that would allow him some quality of life. He would be able to walk, most probably with a pronounced limp, for the rest of his days. He would maybe even be able to manage a bit of golf. But as smart as his new knee joint was, its bag of tricks would not extend to top-flight cricket.

And it was the leg that was the only permanent casualty of his disease and subsequent treatment. His body had responded to the chemotherapy. The tumour had not spread beyond the original site. The surgery had done its job in containing the contamination. The chemo had then swept through, ensuring that any fledgling cancerous cells that had gone undetected were wiped out before they could implant elsewhere. It had also helped that Lythe had enormous confidence in his surgeon Gary French and oncologist David Porter.

Their respective teams had been instrumental in making Lythe as comfortable as he could have been given the circumstances. When it emerged that the cancer had not spread and that Lythe had responded well to the treatment, his medical team exhaled a cautious sigh of relief. They would continue to monitor their man for the next five years. The signs were good, however, that the disease had beaten a hasty retreat.

Lythe's young body would in time recover from the debilitating effects of the chemotherapy. The good cells would regenerate and his strength would return. But the leg was a whole different story. There had been many rotund and supremely unathletic cricket stars. There was in fact a period where it seemed cricketers could only be taken seriously if their girth was every bit as impressive as those who earned a living playing darts. There was a huge difference, though, between a gifted but lardy player and one who was trying to get by on what was effectively half a leg.

To even think about playing first-class cricket was preposterous. To even think he would be able to play cricket at any level was bordering on the insane. He could only walk with crutches. The tiny bit of muscle that was left in his leg had tried to knit back on to the scar tissue and the metal rod. The knee joint would take some time to get used to. Lythe's immediate goal was to get rid of the crutches. Being able to stand and move unsupported would be enormous progress. Even getting to that basic level was going to be a challenge.

Lythe would need to spend hundreds of painful hours in the gym, pushing endless weights for microscopic muscle gains. There would be walking sessions in the swimming pool and in time he would cycle to try and regain a semblance of normality in the ravaged leg. His surgery and treatment had effectively been hell. His rehabilitation had the feel of time in purgatory.

What kept Lythe going was the belief that at some point he would arrive in his own personal heaven. What shape or form that might be, he couldn't be too sure. One thing he did know was that it wouldn't be a heaven where everyone wore cricket whites. Instead, they would all be wearing suits and ties as Lythe made a life-changing decision to study law when he came out of hospital.

'I had started a sports and exercise degree and I guess I went into it for selfish reasons. I was so into sport and I thought it would help with my own training. But I really didn't want to do it as a career. I always had it in my mind that I was going to play sport as a career. I was a teenager so you dream. But after my treatment that had to be rethought. I wanted to study and I wanted to do something that would allow me to work in a number of different areas. The change in direction was one of the big positives.'

The switch to studying law gave Lythe an alternative passion on which he could focus. It didn't necessarily fill the void left by cricket. Nothing would ever do that. What it did do was help him see there was more to life than sport. Coming to that realisation diluted the impact of his cancer. It made him less likely to be angry because he could see that the disease had not robbed him of everything. He had a wonderful, loving, supportive family and good friends. He had a good brain in his head and he had a potentially rewarding and lucrative career awaiting him. And he had his health. That wasn't something he was taking for granted any more. He was alive and there would be more than a few occasions in his early post-treatment life when he took the time to remind himself of that hugely significant fact.

It hadn't escaped Lythe's notice that another talented young Aucklander, Cameron Duncan, had also been diagnosed with osteosarcoma towards the end of the millennium. Duncan, who earned national fame by making a powerful short film, didn't survive. Lythe knew he couldn't be mad about the injustice of losing his sporting career. There had been much more at stake than tossing a leather ball with a bamboozling spin on it. By 2001 he knew all that. And with that knowledge there came a little contentment. He'd been lucky and luck was not the sort of commodity he wanted to get blasé about.

His disposition was also helped by the fact that his leg was getting stronger. Hard work was netting Lythe results. His leg, once so feeble and useless, was responding to the constant exercise. Lythe still wasn't going to win too many 100 metre races, but he was becoming more mobile. His leg had become strong enough for him to play social cricket. And it really was social cricket. He could bowl off a two-step run up and he could hobble between the wickets. His motivation for playing, however, wasn't about results and performance. It was about being part of a team again and enjoying the camaraderie. Well, that was what it was about at first. But in time his ambition gradually evolved.

The incredible thing about Lythe was that he never closed his mind to the potential of what he could achieve. He never fully accepted that as a result of the surgery to his leg, all doors had been slammed in his face. It wasn't that he was fuming away with a desire to prove the world wrong. He didn't set out to be the hero who succeeded in the face of the most severe adversity. It really was a simple case of not making categorical decisions about what he could and couldn't achieve. The situation was fluid. Time, so the cliché goes, is a great healer. He learned not to rule anything out as what seemed impossible six months ago started to feel achievable. As long as the leg continued to respond and improve, he could shift his level of expectation every few weeks.

And so it was that there came a point when he became mobile enough to start thinking beyond social cricket. His leg could support a decent bowling action and it could just about get him between the wickets quickly enough to no longer be considered a liability. Posted at slip he could field without having to chase. It was all still a bit of a struggle, but he felt he could get by at the next level without embarrassing himself or letting down his team-mates.

His old club side, Auckland University, was happy to welcome him back at the start of 2002. They were in trouble and Lythe was worth his place in the team. So much so, in fact, he was asked to be captain. It meant that in just over a year, he had progressed way beyond where he thought possible. His initial plan was to get himself walking without crutches. That progressed to being able to play social cricket. Now he was able to play club cricket. It was still preposterous to think he could go even higher, but that couldn't stop the frustration within Lythe. Things had happened fast and he became impatient to jump to the next stage. He wanted more than just club cricket.

'At times when I was in the gym I thought, why am I doing this? I kept thinking, is it worth it? There was not a week that went by that I wasn't doing something on my leg. That is still true today. It is frustrating pushing piddly weights. I kept pushing on, though, and it kept coming back to the perspective thing. I read about Cameron Duncan and it was so sad he didn't come through it. And often I do think about that when I'm getting anxious and say, hey, it is not that bad. I would often remind myself that I am lucky to be alive and playing at all and I tried to enjoy it.

'But I couldn't do what I wanted to do and playing at club level wasn't going to be enough. I was getting wound up and thinking, why me? And if this hadn't happened I would have been here and here. It was stupid stuff. I had a couple of years like that. I knew I had the ability to do it but that I couldn't because of the physical constraints.'

Lythe's parents looked on, forever amazed at the progress their son was making. While Lythe hadn't once stopped to give himself a hearty pat on the back for far exceeding all initial expectations, his parents and family and friends who had been with him through the journey were simply gob-smacked that he was playing cricket at any level. Perhaps Lythe's parents had better absorbed the reality of what they had been dealing with. Their thought processes had gone along very different lines from their son's. When they heard about his cancer, all they wanted was for their son to live. And then when that goal was achieved and the medics detailed the likely extent of Lythe's post-operative mobility, his parents took the view that the whole issue was not up for debate.

Lythe's mother, Mary, says: 'At the beginning we were waiting for a whole month while the biopsy was sent off to the States. They said it was very rare and he probably could die. I was preparing myself. Then they were adamant he wouldn't be able to walk. They said he would maybe be able to play golf. But he would never run again.

'We were always guided by Tim's strength and serenity. He had a very mature approach to the whole thing. There was no histrionics or him going wild and blaming anybody. It was quite harrowing when he was having the chemotherapy because he was in a dark hole, really. That was difficult because there is no way you can cheer anyone up when they are having chemo and it is making them sick. I guess we were always there for him and he always knew that.

'He saw the whole thing more as a bit of a hitch and he seemed to hang on to that dream of playing for the Aces even when he was told he would only just be able to walk. We never said, don't be so silly. We had the attitude that he would reach his potential at whatever level and he should just go for it. The surgeon was surprised each time he did something.

'Tim was the one who organised the brothers and cousins in the social team. His buttock and leg were completely wasted and there was nothing there. Everything had to reform and attach to this piece of metal. I secretly thought, "He won't get very far." He changed course academically to study law. He could have done his sports science degree but he said he didn't want to be a cripple telling top athletes what to do. It was only more recently that I said, "What did you think about dying?" And he said, "I just didn't think about it."'

Lythe simply refused to acknowledge any potential outcomes he didn't like the sound of. It was classic ignore it and it will go away. But it helped him stay focused on what he wanted to achieve. It allowed him to believe he could achieve the impossible. Keeping the cold facts at bay was not such a bad strategy. He needed to be driven by emotion. If he thought about the reality it would close off both his heart and mind to his true potential.

When he assessed the facts about his cricket ability, what he knew for sure was that he was taking wickets at club level. He was by no means a sympathy selection – he was there because he was good enough. His leg would never recover to its pre-surgery state. The mobility and strength would be restricted forever. Yet, there was clearly still a window of opportunity for Lythe. His physical limitations could be circumnavigated. So what that he was a bit awkward as he ran in to bowl. He had still managed to fashion an effective action. It would not be a huge drama that he would miss out on a few quick singles whenever he batted, and there are plenty of cricketers who only ever field at slip.

As he took in the facts, it began to dawn on him that he could shift the frontier of ambition to the next level. As ridiculous as it seemed, he could salvage the dying embers of his sporting dream. He was fortunate that he had a surgeon who was capable of seeing the big picture, too. His knee would not last forever. At some stage it would need to be replaced.

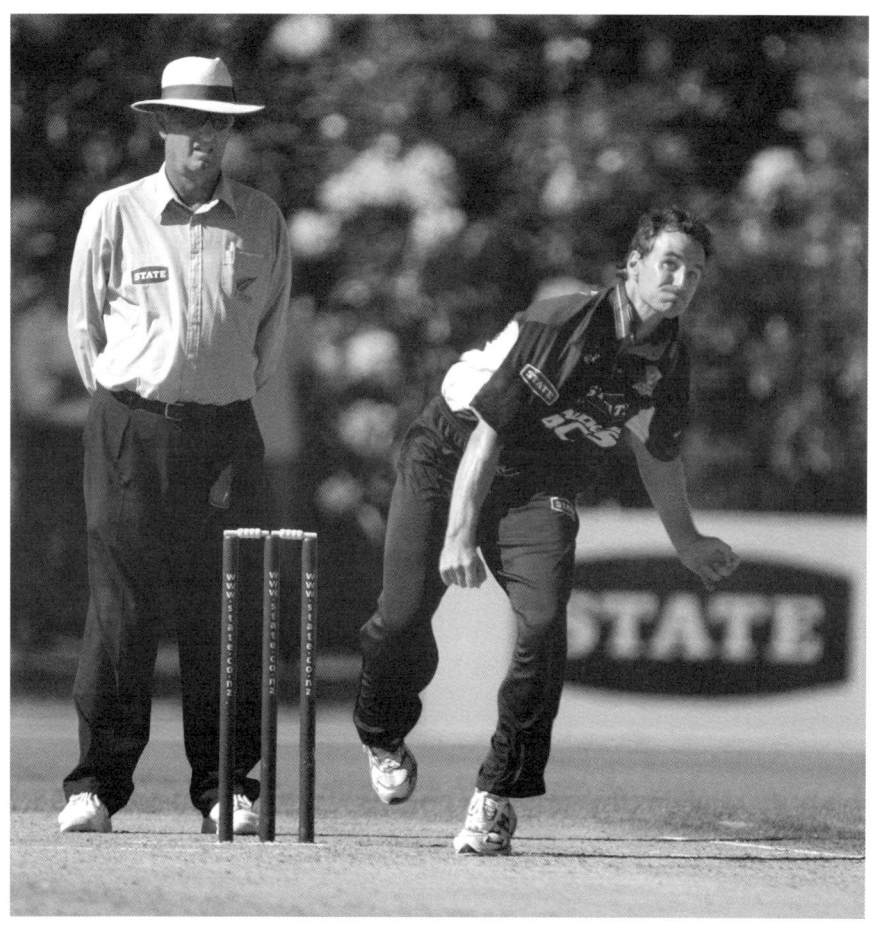

Tim Lythe in action for Auckland Aces against Central Stags in the State Shield, January 2006. *Tim Hales, Photosport*

But thankfully the surgeon saw there was no need to be precious about the joint. The window to play cricket was now. If that meant exposing the joint to excessive wear and tear and having to replace it sooner than scheduled, so be it. Lythe was cruising along nicely with his study. A career in law would always be there for him. Professional cricket wouldn't.

'It wasn't a flick of the switch. It was more gradual. My leg became stronger and I got more mobile so my cricket got better. It was very gradual over three seasons. I was taking wickets and I was going okay. I started to think after a while that maybe I could do something and I got into the Auckland B team. I was lucky that the surgeon was very understanding and he pretty much said go for it. I remember he said, "Life is not a dress rehearsal," and I loved that quote and still do. They continue to be my favourite motivational words. I think after he said that, there was definitely a period where I thought, "Let's give this a crack and if it doesn't work there is no drama." '

And that is exactly what he did. He continued to push himself to breaking point and he continued to take wickets at club and Auckland B level. And most important of all, he continued to believe that his chance would come. That's all he wanted – just one game for Auckland to say he had done it. No one could ever take that away from him.

His faith was severely tested. His path was being blocked by Brooke Walker, who was not only a fine leg spinner, he was also Auckland's captain. There was only room for one spinner and Lythe had his moments when he thought about chucking the towel in. Just fleeting instances when he felt he was banging his head against a brick wall that was never going to tumble.

He had started work with the law firm Minter Ellison. His career was taking off. Did he really need first-class cricket anyway? It would derail the momentum he was building in his law work. As those thoughts became a little more frequent towards the 2004-2005 season, he got the news he had been waiting for.

'Brooke Walker retired. The last few seasons I had been sitting in behind him and that provided other frustrations as I was never going to break in. He was a quality player and captain. I actually contemplated giving it away a few times. But when he retired I thought that would be my window. I didn't actually expect a contract so that was a bonus and it provided a bigger window as it said, "You are in our thoughts, now go and make the most of it." '

There was a fairytale ending after all. Lythe, the man who would never walk again, was contracted to play first-class cricket alongside the country's finest. How could this be? Well, according to Auckland coach Mark O'Donnell it is because Lythe is a very fine cricketer himself. 'He is one of the first names we put down on the team sheet,' says O'Donnell. 'We knew the full extent of Tim's leg surgery and we had no concerns with that. When Brooke retired we offered Tim a contract and left the decision up to him whether he took it. We knew he would have some limitations with his leg, but we made it clear to him that we would only use him in the four-day games and not the one-day games. It was a pretty easy choice to offer him the contract.'

Ask Lythe the same question about how it was that he was able to make such a spectacular comeback and he offers only pragmatism in response. He puts it down to hard work, belief, ability and a little bit of luck. He is right, yet that doesn't seem enough. It's way too understated. Plenty of other people have applied themselves in the same way and got nowhere near as far as Lythe. He has managed to get to the top after having had half his leg removed. But he is a reluctant hero. He deals in pragmatism because he genuinely believes he did nothing special. He simply adapted after he was dealt a bad hand. It is for others to provide more objective accounts of what he has achieved. His mother does a pretty good job of summarising what most observers who know the facts believe.

'It is a miracle just to see Tim running on the pitch. We watch him play and we just can't believe where he has come from in five years. He just kept going and I can remember looking at him one day and saying, "Tim, which leg did you have done?" Most people don't know he's got several metal bits inside his leg. They know he has had something wrong with his knee but a lot of sportsmen have had that. Some of the top selectors, even though they have read articles on Tim, they still haven't taken on board they have effectively got a disabled player and he really shouldn't be there.

'We laugh and I say to him that he ought to be in the Paralympics. It is not normal for someone with his disability to be playing elite sport. His peer group who didn't go through it with him don't realise what form of disability it is. He doesn't ever excuse himself for it. He never says anything is too tough. He wouldn't want to play if they were just being nice to him.'

He needn't worry about that. Lythe is in the team on merit, as he proved when he came in as a night watchman in Auckland's first State Shield game in the 2005-2006 season and knocked 63 runs. His bowling figures weren't too shabby either, with Lythe claiming two wickets for 46 runs. The cap he had craved since the summer of 1999 was finally his. Yet, in typical Lythe fashion, there was no emotional meltdown. He didn't walk off the field in Napier with the sense he had fulfilled his destiny. He walked off reasonably chuffed with his own efforts but utterly dissatisfied that the team had drawn. It wasn't about him. It was always about the team and getting the win they needed to challenge at the right end of the competition.

Once again his objectives had changed. For so long he had dreamed of winning a solitary cap. But when that goal appeared almost certain to be achieved back in July 2005 when he signed his contract, he wanted much more than a single appearance.

'When I was trying to break into the team I kept thinking, "If I could have just played one game for Auckland no one could have taken that away from me." I just wanted to be able to say I had played for Auckland. Now I have got that, I have widened my horizons. Maybe my leg can keep getting stronger. There is definitely a cap on my physical capacity but I'll just have to keep pushing it to find out where that is.

'If I could get a few seasons for Auckland I would be satisfied with that. If I could play a number of games and contribute – that is what I would like to be remembered for. I would like to win a few games and be remembered as a good team man.

'Sometimes I get wound up and I say to myself, relax and just enjoy the moment. It is a huge bonus to be where I am. It is at those times that I think where I have come from and that I never should have been able to play at all, let alone at this level. But at other times I think I have done all the hard work and I need to give a little more. I tend to think that I will push this to the limit because that is the person I am. How many people get the chance to do this?

'I kind of hate the fact people bring up my cancer and my leg. I have got a number of team-mates and people I play against who are not aware of it. I don't want to be judged differently. I am a cricketer. Judge me as a cricketer and for what I do for the team. I don't think I have done anything that any other Kiwi wouldn't have done. All I have done is tried to live and do the things that I love. What else was I going to do? I had a lot of luck along the way. I didn't say, "I am going to come out of this as something special."

'I tend to keep asking myself how far I can go in the game. Realistically, I don't think I could play for New Zealand. One, I don't think I'm good enough. That could be a confidence thing. But there is the mobility issue as well. Playing for New Zealand is a dream but I don't think it is a realistic goal. But maybe I can keep on improving.'

Maybe making the Black Caps is a step too far for Lythe. But given the way he has shown scant regard for reality in the past, only the very brave would bet against him one day playing test cricket.

Tim Lythe juggles his time between the law firm Minter Ellison and the Auckland Aces where he is a contracted player. Having played for Auckland Under-19s in 1999, Lythe played his first full game for the Aces in 2005 and scored 63 runs against Central Districts and took two wickets for 46 runs. He is 25 and lives in Auckland.

9

AARON SLIGHT

World Superbikes 1992-2000

Study only the raw statistics of Aaron Slight's racing career and they give the impression 2000 was his most disappointing season as a world superbike rider. As one-time British Prime Minister Benjamin Disraeli is believed to have said, there are lies, damn lies and statistics. Slight finished eighth in 2000, his lowest placing in nine seasons of competition. What the record books don't state, though, is that in 2000, Slight missed the first six races. That didn't necessarily need to be catastrophic in terms of his final placing. There was still enough time upon his return to garner championship points and make a charge up the ladder.

But Slight missed those races because he was recovering from brain surgery to have a life-threatening lesion removed. The surgery was major. The 2000 season should have bypassed Slight completely. It should have been a year of rehabilitation and the notion of winning world superbike races is not one that should ever have entered his head. There should have been no trace of Slight in the record books. He had not only missed three meets, he was also struggling with serious mental and physical fatigue. He returned to racing having done virtually no testing and having not been on his bike at all for the better part of four months.

The concentration and mental endurance required to be a challenger at world superbikes is enormous. Make one small mistake and you can drop several places in a flash. Make one moderate mistake and you can be flying off your bike. Given the severity of his operation and subsequent rehabilitation, Slight should have been parked in front of the box for the remainder of the season, watching his compatriots slug it out from the comfort of his home. He wasn't though.

Three months after being discharged, Slight was caning his bike round the Donnington Park track in the UK. The racing fraternity watched in awe. They knew what it took to compete at this level and they knew that far from being a season of shame, 2000 was possibly Slight's greatest achievement.

It was an astonishing comeback. His situation only a few months before he raced at Donnington was desperate. He had effectively suffered a stroke at the tender age of 34. That would seem about as bad as it could get and if he had quit his sport on the spot, citing an emotional breakdown as the cause, everyone would have understood.

But Slight's reaction was the polar opposite. Instead of being plunged into a tumultuous emotional torment, he slipped into altogether more placid territory. On hearing the news he had a two-centimetre bleed in his brain, Slight felt only relief. It was relief that at last he had proof he wasn't going mad. As he had suspected for the better part of the previous 12 months, there was something seriously wrong with him. There was also an element of relief that there was a chance he might be able to resume his racing career.

That might seem like false bravado. To only feel relief appears almost disrespectful to what was a mighty serious ailment. There must have been more to it. Surely Slight was panicking when he was told there was a problem with his brain that could kill him? Fear must have played a role. Both his career and his life were on the line. But this wasn't so different to any other day. His life was on the line every time he sat on his motorbike and raced. His machine was capable of speeds in excess of 300 km/h. Even with all the safety gear, it doesn't make for a pretty sight when riders come off at that speed. Death was a possible, albeit unlikely, outcome every time he raced. Facing up to his diagnosis wasn't so different. He was pretty used to the looming threat, so he'd learned not to be fearful.

The prospect of his career ending was, maybe bizarrely, potentially more of a concern. He wasn't ready for that, and the sacrifices he had made to get to the top of his sport were too great to have anyone other than himself call time on his career. The battle to the world circuit had been a tough one. For a start, Slight had grown up in Masterton – a town not recognised as the epicentre of elite motorcycling. There were no local heroes inspiring him and nothing directly linking him to the world circuit.

Nor were the Slight family's financial resources equipped to deal with the constant pounding exerted by the sport. Racing bikes is not cheap. As a young motocross rider, Slight was the kid who had to get through the season with just one set of tyres. He was the kid racing in his dad's old scooter helmet and work boots. The struggle was relentless. When he first tried to cut it as a professional, he lived in a friend's Sydney apartment that was so small it could have easily been mistaken for a toaster.

Slight put up with the hardships because he loved racing. There was nothing he wanted to do more than get on a motorbike and ride it as fast as he possibly could. If winning races required him to live a lifestyle some way short of salubrious then so be it. He would not be moaning.

Given the size of his emotional and financial investment in the sport, the thought of losing it all should have terrified him. But while it might seem innocuous by comparison, Slight felt the hand injury he incurred in 1990 was much more of an ordeal than having his head cut open and a piece of brain removed. His career, so he was told, was over before it had ever really begun. He defied the odds in 1990 and that is why he was confident that, 10 years later, he could do it again.

He knew that his interpretation of impossible differed from most other people's. He knew that as long as there was a sliver of hope he could return to the track that would be enough. His dedication to the sport would always see him triumph. Hard work, belief in himself and a confidence that he could succeed would enable him to overcome any adversity.

He knew all that in 2000 because he had learned it in 1990. He was in his first year racing for a Kawasaki factory team in Japan when he came

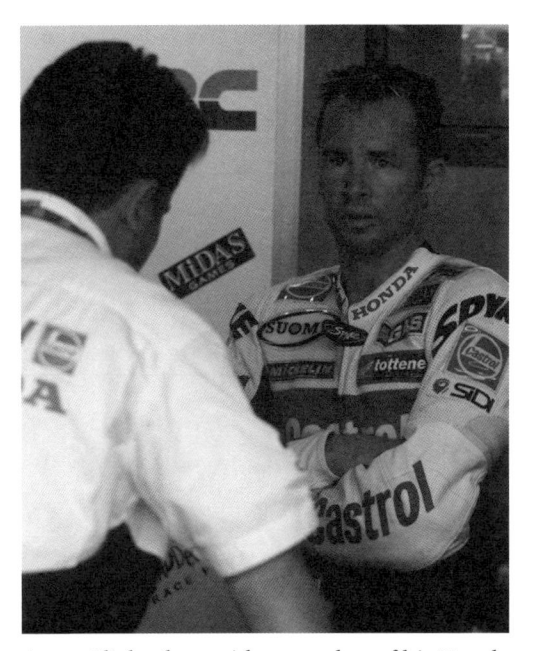

Aaron Slight chats with a member of his Honda team. *Graeme Brown*

off his bike. It wouldn't have been a particularly dramatic crash but for the fact he got his right hand caught under his wheel. He lost his little finger and destroyed the tendons in his other fingers. If he had been an accountant or a lawyer, the situation wouldn't have been disastrous. The surgeons could restore his hand to the point where it would be able to function well enough to get a pass mark in most basic activities. Typing and writing would be achievable, if a little laboured. He would be able to get by around the house. But his ambition extended far beyond that. He wanted to race enormously powerful motorbikes. To do that, his right hand would have to be earning more than pass marks. It would be charged with controlling the throttle and brake – vital functions. He needed a feathery touch to excel in a sport where races are won and lost by thousandths of seconds.

When he returned to New Zealand after his accident, the surgeon struggled to see how Slight's ravaged appendage would ever recover enough to fulfil its destiny. As Slight remembers: 'The accident in Japan, to me, was more dramatic than having the brain thing. Because my hand got stuck under the bike, I ground the back of it away. I flew back to New Zealand to have it fixed in the Hutt Hospital. Most people thought that would be the end of my career. It was my second year of being paid.

'I had surgery done by a guy called Dr Glasson. He was a burns specialist. He took a big knife to the inside of my forearm and took off a donor site. He took a bone out of there as well and reconstructed my little finger. The top of my hand had gone. He also reconstructed my tendons so I only have two tendons that operate my fingers. My index finger and the one next to it work together and the other two work together.

'It happened in June and my big goal was to ride before the end of the year. If I hadn't, they would have let me go. I was probably feeding my team a bit of a line that I was all right. But it was more hope at that stage. I had no idea. I was living in Masterton and I was travelling about 100 km over the Rimutakas four times a week for physio after the operation. It would be an hour and a quarter there and an hour and a quarter back. It was very tough on my hand. During the operation, they stitched the tendons on my hand and then they glued and healed. We were trying to move these tendons under the skin so you are almost tearing the flesh away as you try to move them. We had to use nitrous oxide most days because the pain was unbearable.'

The clock was ticking. Slight had to get back on his bike before the end of the season. It's a cut-throat business and corporations need more than just verbal assurance that a rider with a bung hand can win races.

He had no choice but to resume riding before the end of the year. His hand was not ready. The agony inflicted by the physio had yielded some improvement. He had more flexibility than anyone initially believed possible. But he was still taking a massive risk.

'The doctor did marvels with my hand and I talked my way back into getting a ride for the rest of the year. But I didn't really have that good a grip and the braking was really a problem for me. The handlebar flopped around in my hand and wiggled away a bit. It wasn't great but I think I had a sixth in the world championship in one of my comeback rides and that was enough to convince them to keep me.'

Slight, though, was not getting carried away when the new contract came through. His position was still tenuous. Sure he could race, but not at the level that would see him become a world-class rider. He would remain in the expendable category with his hand the way it was. Soon enough the next best thing would come along and before he could protest, he would be yesterday's man. He had scrambled a recovery of sorts. To preserve his dreams he needed to convince his doctor to once more whip out his trusty blade.

'I was lucky that I had a doctor who was so committed to getting me back. If you have a bung hand it doesn't really matter to them. You can go back and be a labourer or whatever. They didn't want to operate again but after I went back to riding the bike, the physiotherapist and I convinced him that they had to.

'At the end of that season I had another operation where they loosened off the tendons. My finger was a bit wrong too, so I took a handlebar in with me and said, "Make my hand fit this." So he did. The minute I woke up from the second operation the doctors said, "Don't stop moving your hand." It sounds disgusting but I woke up and started moving my fingers and blood and shit were going everywhere.

'It was about getting my hand right. You have got to be at the top of your game at that level. You really do need to be an athlete to ride these bikes. I won an eight-hour race once by 0.008 of a second. Every lap has to be spot-on. When you are riding your bike your heart is at 90 per cent. Your arms, your back, your legs and chest are knackered.

'If I got my hand right to ride a motorbike then it was going to be right to do a lot of other things as well. If I had said, "Thanks a lot for the surgery, I'm going home," I would have had a stuffed hand for whatever I ended up doing. I wanted it to be as good as I could get it.

'When I got back the next season I won the Australian championship and the Pan Pacific championship. I won just about every race I started. I was so fired up that I was having a second chance. It gave me confidence to go fast when I was in control and when I didn't feel like that, I wouldn't bow to peer pressure. I would be confident to say, "It is wrong and I am going to finish second today." I got a lot of confidence. I was mentally a lot stronger. It made me realise that I had been riding a motorbike flat out all the time.'

It was a hungrier, more confident Slight who came back in 1991. From being a potential career-ender, Slight's hand injury became the catalyst for a much improved performance. The following year he was signed to race in the world superbike championship. Only 18 months after having to contemplate ending his career he was beating the very biggest names in the sport. The boy from Masterton wasn't pausing for breath. The best way to prove his hand was not an issue was to win races. And that is exactly what he did for the next seven years.

In 1992, his debut season in world superbikes, he finished sixth. Between 1993 and 1998 Slight finished either second or third in the world championship. It was usually only those riders who had the luxury of sitting atop a twin cylinder Ducati that beat him. The curiosity of the world championship rules meant four-cylinder machines were restricted to 750 cc, while twin-cylinder machines could run with 1000 cc engines. Neither of the two teams Slight raced for – Honda and Kawasaki – made four-cylinder machines, which left him having to battle against the bigger engines of Carl Fogarty and Troy Corser. Slight managed to win his share of individual races, but over the course of a season, his bike couldn't match the consistency of the Ducatis.

There was frustration, for sure, that an elusive world championship kept proving beyond him. He was in it to win it. It was nice that he was being paid more than handsomely for his troubles. It was nice that as a consequence of his wealth, he was able to live in the tax haven of Monaco – the chosen playground of the rich and famous. But he wasn't doing it for the cash. He wanted the glory of winning. That was why he had lived in a shoebox in Sydney. That was why he had spent a curious year racing in Japan where he spent most of his time away from the track sitting in the team owner's garage showroom as if he were some rare zoo exhibit. And then there was the agony of rehabilitating his hand. That pain had been endured for a reason – so he could go on and be the best bike racer in the world.

Maybe 1999 would be his year. But once the season started Slight suspected otherwise. He couldn't put his finger on it, but he knew he wasn't quite right. His reactions felt as if they had lost their razor sharpness. His vision wasn't quite as acute as it should have been. He was suffering from a lethargy he had never previously encountered. It wasn't dramatic, he just felt a bit off his top form. His performances suffered accordingly. There was no major collapse in form, just a gradual decline.

As the season went on his deterioration gathered pace. He began to suffer blinding headaches. The tiredness got worse, the vision more blurry. His frustration was amplified by the continued failure of the blood tests and CT scans to pick up anything. He finished fourth in the championship in 1999. It was still a solid achievement, but it was the worst finish for Slight since his rookie season. He was in his early 30s and this should have been his optimum window of opportunity. Experience in his sport was vital. It takes riders years to learn when to attack and when to consolidate. The art of concentrating for such prolonged periods also improves with age. Slight should have been at his racing peak.

But instead, by early 2000, he was beside himself. Everything had become a chore. He was feeling awful and no one could tell him why. His world couldn't stop to be fixed. He was testing for the new season, his vision so impaired by now that he was riding his bike at 300 km/h without really being able to see where he was going. He knew then he had to get off the track and get some sort of answer as to what the hell was wrong with him.

'I got on the bike at Eastern Creek in Sydney and did about 10 laps and I couldn't actually focus. My lap times were about six seconds slower than everyone else. At this level, if you are not on the pace after two or three laps, something is not right. I came in and said to the guys, "I don't know what is wrong." I couldn't focus and it got worse and worse that day. I said I was going to hurt myself. I had never thought that before. I had to make a call. Rather than swing my leg over and prove I could go fast, I didn't know what was happening. I had really bad double vision so I rang my doctor in New Zealand.

'I said, "I know you have done all these tests but I know I have a problem." She sent over all my reports to a doctor in Sydney. She had the file and it was pretty thick. On the very last page there was a handwritten note saying, "We have taken no imagery of his head." I had had a CT scan but never an MRI scan.

'So I drove myself to the hospital. I had one eye closed so I could see where I was going. I got there and they put me through the MRI machine. They said it would take about 15 minutes and I was there for 45, so I knew something was up. These machines are really claustrophobic and horrible, but while I was lying there I actually felt some relief. I was thinking that, at long last, they were actually going to find out what was wrong with me. When I came out they said they had found a two-centimetre bleed on the brain. My reaction was, "What do we do?" I had racing in a few weeks' time.

'The guy I wanted to see came back from California and gave me three options. He said we could leave it and hopefully it would go away. I didn't really like the sound of that for obvious reasons. He mentioned laser and radiation treatment but they prefer to use that when the lesion is less than one centimetre. The third option was to open up my head and take the lesion out. I said, "What are we waiting for? Let's get on with it." The next night he operated.'

Slight didn't bother fretting about it too much. He had spent the last year or so doing exactly that. Now was the time to start thinking about the future as he could at last see himself returning to the track in full working order. The surgery carried a risk. They were meddling with his brain, after all, and the lesion was in an awkward position – it was close to his brain stem. But he had confidence in the surgeon and faith in his own ability to recover. There was no need for panic.

'It was a huge relief. At the end of the year I was almost suicidal, thinking, "What's fucking wrong with me? People don't believe me that I'm not well." It was a really bad time. I would say to people, "I'm so tired and I don't feel well," and they would say, "No problem, it is all in your head, you will be okay." It was all in my fucking head, all right.

'It was another lesson. I listened to my body and I knew my body. I don't think a normal person would have known there was something up until the bleed. When you are working on a motorcycle and you are talking about splits of seconds, you know when you are not at your best. There was something stopping me from being my best. It was like I was losing that sixth sense when I was riding. I could be going 320 km/h down a straight and know that someone was coming up on my shoulder without looking. I was losing that. I was having to look.

'No one knows how or when the lesion happened. But I believe it had been putting a small bit of pressure on my brain for some time. We were testing at Phillip Island just before Eastern Creek. I was going okay.

I wasn't the fastest but I wasn't the slowest either. I went for a swim in the surf with my mechanics and I can remember diving in and not feeling well. I hit the wave and thought, I'm over this. I'm getting out. As I walked out I was looking into the sun and the pain was severe. I knew something was really up then.

'They did an angiogram and I realised how dangerous the surgery was. I had to sign a disclaimer because there was a risk of death or paralysis. This is where they put a catheter into your groin and then they pump dye into your brain so they can take a photo of it. The surgery almost took my ear off. They cut from the bottom of my sideburn straight up for about five centimetres, then across for about five centimetres and then five centimetres down behind my ear. They lifted the skull out and then removed the lesion. Because it was at the base of my brain stem it was affecting my fine motor skills and was affecting my vision because it was pushing on my optic nerve. That was one of the things I was worried about, so I said to the doctor, "I'm going in as Aaron Slight. Will I come out as him?"

'He said that it shouldn't affect my personality or anything like that. That was a bit of a relief. It took about four hours. When the doctor put the skull back together he usually just glued it. But because I was going back racing he screwed and plated my head.'

And racing was exactly what Slight intended to do. He knew he could recover. He'd been through all that before. Brain surgery was not going to be enough to convince him to give up. He had unfinished business on the track. Seeing the world title elude his grasp was something he had come to hate. There was still enough time for him to win that coveted world championship. Winning in 2000 was out of the question. But doing so in the next couple of years was realistic. At 34 he still had enough time.

The great unknown, however, was whether his brain would recover enough to allow him his last chance at glory. His problem had been fixed in the sense that his life was no longer under threat and he would no longer be afflicted by blinding headaches and impaired vision. The doctors were reasonably sure he would, in time, be living a normal life. But whether he would be able to resume his career in world superbikes was an entirely different matter. That, they didn't know.

It's a legal requirement for everyone who has brain surgery to surrender his or her driving licence for a year. The law is in place because there is an element of unpredictability attached to all brain surgery. The brain is such a powerful and finely balanced piece of machinery that any tampering with it can have dramatic consequences.

Quite often those consequences are not apparent until the rehabilitation process is in full swing. Slight would not particularly want to be travelling at 300 km/h and only then discover that his brain had developed some idiosyncrasies. His reactions needed to be instinctive and immediate to get back racing. He was going to have to be able to get through hour after hour of intense concentration. The rigour of superbikes is just as much mental as it is physical. If he couldn't keep focused for the duration of a race, his safety would become a major issue. The surgeon who opened up Slight's head couldn't promise that his patient would be up to the demands of continuing with his chosen career. All he could be sure about was that Slight would be very tired for the first few months of his recovery. He also knew that Slight would struggle to concentrate on specific tasks for any length of time and that he would most likely become frustrated and disillusioned more easily than he had in his pre-surgery life. How quickly those side effects would subside, he couldn't be sure.

Not that any of this made a blind bit of difference to Slight. The doctors could hum and haw and talk about ifs and buts and pots and pans. He kept his focus much more streamlined. He would return – end of story.

'I had a really quick recovery. Once again, because I was focused, that was all I was going to do. I had a plan. I didn't get up in the morning and mope around. I had to get on with it. I woke up in intensive care. Before going in I had to hand over my gold card and pay for it. I signed away three days in intensive care and seven days in the hospital. I was out within four. I only spent 14 hours in intensive care and another three days in hospital.

'I was staying in a B&B close to the hospital. Things to me seemed to be going really slow. I can remember one day sitting by the pool and I sat there all day. And at the end of the day I thought, "This is really weird." I had been sitting there all day not thinking. And then I thought, "If I had not been thinking, what had I actually been thinking?" Then I started to think, "If I'm thinking that then maybe I'm okay." The thing with the brain is it controls everything so you feel like you want to cut your head off and give it a rest. But you can't, and the only thing you can do is nothing when you are awake. You don't realise how much thinking you have to do to do something.

'My first outing after the operation was to a coffee shop but once I got there the noise of the traffic was unbearable and I couldn't be there. I came home after two weeks and returned to my farm in Masterton. I was riding my little bike round the farm and came off and hit my head. When someone opens up your head you are supposed to hand in your driving licence. I didn't do that and whether it was right or wrong, driving and riding were part of my physio.

'At the same time I was on to my team in England asking what I had to do to get back. I started to realise that if I could ride within 12 weeks I would be able to ride at Donnington Park. That was the fourth round of the championship. My doctor had given me clearance to ride after three months. So I rang him back and said, "Can you make it 12 weeks?" He agreed. I went to Donnington and I had 10 laps the day before so they could assess me. They said, "Yes, you are cleared," and I rode in the race.

'I wasn't scared when I went back. The brain thing was a natural disaster. This was always going to happen. It wouldn't have mattered if I was a bike rider or worked in McDonalds, I was always going to have a stroke. It didn't put me off racing. It just gave me the goal to get back into it. I only had a couple of years left anyway so if I didn't like it I could always go and do something else. In retrospect I did come back too early but that was the only way I would keep my job. If I had taken a year off, I wouldn't have had a job next year. Also, there was the whole stigma about my brain. If I didn't ride, people wouldn't believe I could. After I came back, I raced every race and finished eighth in the championship.'

His wife, Megan, was there as always when Slight returned. She had watched her husband since his brain surgery and realised that he absolutely had to get back into his sport. His racing defined him. He wouldn't have been happy if he had never even tried to get back on the bike.

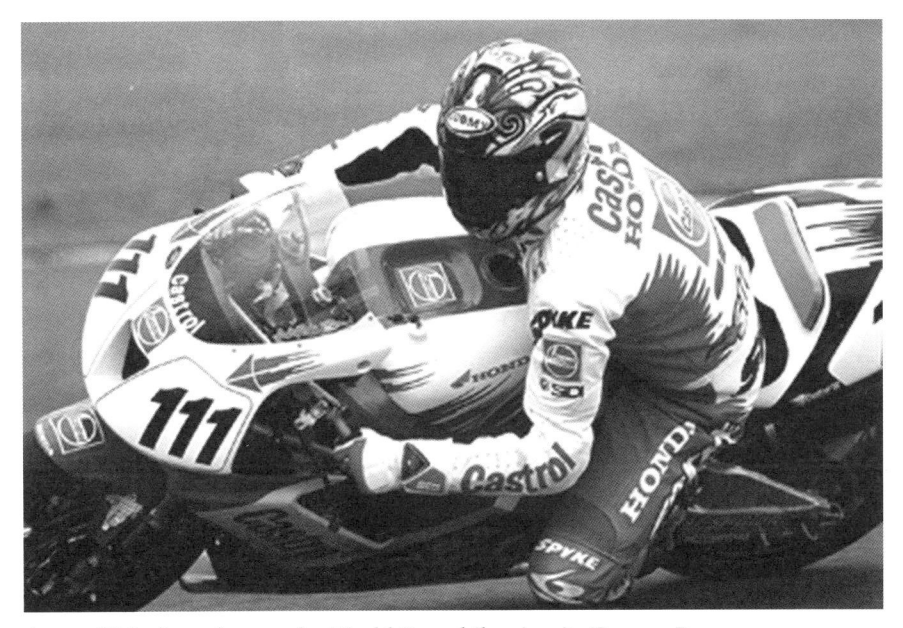

Aaron Slight in action on the World Superbike circuit. *Graeme Brown*

'It did occur to me at first that this was a pretty good opportunity for Aaron to get out,' she says. 'Some professional athletes struggle with the best way to get out and sometimes an injury is the easiest way. But then I realised how much motivation it had given him trying to get back. It was an absolute struggle for him and it was an amazing achievement that he returned. It was a miracle that he wasn't just racing, but that he was also doing really well.

'The best part I think was the way the fans reacted to him when he returned. Everywhere we went he was so well supported and the crowds cheered for him. It reminded you on a daily basis what he had been through.'

Slight had done the unthinkable. The romance of his achievement was lost on his team bosses, however. They didn't get all misty-eyed at Slight's comeback. Instead, they showed the ruthless nature of the sport and didn't renew his contract. They told Slight just before he went out to race in the final meet of the season at Brands Hatch. That year, 2000, as it turned out, was Slight's farewell season. It was a bitter pill to swallow at the time. Not made any easier by the fact that Slight's Honda team-mate,

Colin Edwards, won the world championship that year. Edwards's victory was proof that the manufacturer had obviously got the bike just right. Slight could only wonder how he might have fared had he been fully fit and had he enjoyed a full testing and racing programme on a machine that was probably the fastest Honda had ever built.

'On one level it was Aaron's best season,' says Megan. 'But on another it was his worst. It was amazing that he had achieved his personal goal of getting back into racing. When you look at it rationally, it was a miracle that he did. But it was bitter-sweet for us because his goal was also to have his contract renewed and it was so disappointing when he lost his job.'

But time, as it so often is, was a great healer. With a bit of space, Slight could see that he had enjoyed a remarkable career. He could see there were plenty of highlights and also that he had been able to bow out on the back of an incredible season. He had fulfilled the showbiz mantra – always leave them wanting more.

'The next year when I was replaced, the Japanese guy who took my place didn't even finish eighth. I was demanding quite big money at the time. That could have been a factor why they didn't renew my contract. I believe that with the Japanese, because of the communication problem, once you are damaged goods you are damaged goods. They didn't know if I was still as good or the same person. You tell someone you have had a brain operation and they immediately think you are a bit weird. I think it was all that plus the fact I only had two years left anyway.

'It was horrific coming back from the brain surgery, so I was distraught that I couldn't go on. It was the way it was done. I had worked for Honda for seven years. They told me at the last meeting I didn't have a contract. By then I couldn't get a ride anywhere else so they virtually retired me. Looking back maybe it was the right thing. But it should have been my choice.

'But I went back to Monaco and wrote my book. That was the first time I had reflected on my career. I was really happy to be in that position. I was happy to walk away from it. I got to reflecting and I realised that I had a great career.'

It took Slight a while to realise he had a great career. He would probably be the only one so slow on the uptake.

Aaron Slight is recognised as one of the best riders ever to have graced the World Superbikes championship and certainly the best rider never to actually win the title. He came second to the Australian rider Troy Corser in 1996 and then missed out in 1998 to the legendary Carl Fogarty. Slight finished third in 1993, 1994, 1995 and 1997. He performed at the peak of the sport's popularity and many dedicated fans still believe his epic encounters with Fogarty and Corser were some of the best the sport has witnessed. After he retired at the end of the 2000 season he switched to racing tour cars in the UK for Peugeot before returning to his home in Masterton in 2005. He continues to advise Honda on various matters.

10

HIKA REID

All Black 1980-1986

The roar of the crowd drifted into Hika Reid's hospital room. He had a sense that something historic was happening at the nearby Waikato Stadium. It was 11 June 2005 and the New Zealand Maori were playing the British Lions.

Reid should have been at the stadium. He was technical adviser for the Maori team. Only a few weeks earlier the plan had been pretty straightforward. He would be in Auckland on Sunday, 27 May to give a presentation to the Maori team before flying out with them to Fiji for a week. The day after the Maori played Fiji in Suva, Reid's beloved Bay of Plenty would have the honour of being the first provincial side to tear into the touring Lions. As the Irish might say, the trip to Fiji was going to be great craic. And once Reid got back, the Maori would head down to Hamilton to play the Lions. After that he was bracing himself to host some old mates from Ireland who were coming out to take in the rest of the Lions tour. It was going to be a magic six weeks or so. Rugby, beers and old mates – most red-blooded males would agree those three ingredients combined make the ultimate entertainment.

But that plan had to be radically altered when towards the end of May, Reid started seeing what looked like a lightning flash in the corner of his left eye. It was irritating to the point of distraction. He had to take himself off to the optometrist. He was diagnosed with a detached retina and had the eye operated on.

But there was something bothering the specialist. There were dark patches behind the eye. He felt they needed to be investigated. Reid was packed off to have his blood tested. No one really made too big a thing of it so he trundled off believing the tests to be nothing more than routine. He was satisfying the needless, precautionary conservatism of a medic who wanted to be sure his own back was covered.

Reid didn't give it another thought. He didn't really have time to worry whether he might be ill. His only thoughts were for his forthcoming rugby odyssey. The next few weeks would have a significant impact on his coaching career. Not only that, having played for the Bay of Plenty 85 times and still being attached to the union as a development officer, he had significant emotion invested in the outcome of what would be one of the biggest games in the Steamers' history.

The same was true of the Maori. Reid had enjoyed peripheral involvement preparing both teams. He was not going to be centre stage if either team pulled off historic victories but the experience would sit well on his CV. It would add just a little more weight to his list of coaching achievements and help nudge forward an already impressive reputation.

So when he got back to his house in Rotorua after his eye operation and subsequent blood tests, Reid ignored the message from the hospital to get in touch immediately. After all, how serious could it be? The specialist had said during the examination, "Don't worry, we don't think it's cancer." It could all wait until after the weekend. Presumably he would live that long.

The next day he drove up to Auckland to speak to the Maori team who were in camp. As a proud Maori, Reid was delighted to be asked. He had the mana to inspire. He was a former All Black and is recognised as being supremely unfortunate to have only won eight test caps. He also in both 1980 and 1983 won the Tom French Cup – the trophy awarded to the year's most outstanding Maori player.

There was more to it than that, though. Reid is also one of the game's good guys, eminently likeable with that easy-going charm that wins him friends wherever he travels. But as he stood in front of the roomful of young men in Auckland, he had an eerie sense things were not as they should be. 'When I had heard the messages they had been leaving on my answerphone, I thought stuff that, I'm still going up to Auckland. But when I started talking to the Maori boys, I was sweating pretty hard,' he recalls. 'I think a lot of the guys just thought I was nervous. But by then I knew there was something wrong.'

Ignoring the messages left by the hospital was the response of a man who had never taken a backward step. Everything in Reid's life had been confronted head-on. He had learned to fend for himself from almost before he could even remember. His father died when he was 18 months old and his mother when he was eight. It made for a tough upbringing. He was loved and cared for by his brother and whanau, but they could never replace the emotional support and guidance of his parents. Without his parents' watchful eyes on him 24/7, it was easy for Reid to slip under the radar. He could have sampled life on the wild side. But Reid battled to steer himself away from the potential trouble it would have been all too easy for him to find.

His rugby life, too, had in a sense been all about overcoming obstacles. He burst on to the test scene in 1980 by scoring a memorable try against Australia. He had been one of the few standouts on the tour but his selection had only come about because the incumbent, Andy Dalton, was injured. Once Dalton recovered, Reid was back on the bench. He sat there too many times between 1981 and 1985, only getting a run on a couple of tours when Dalton was unavailable. It was frustrating for a man who had obvious talent that would have earned him a hatful of caps in any other era. It was also frustrating because Reid had worked so damned hard to get himself into that position.

When Sean Fitzpatrick came to prominence in 1986 and effectively relegated Reid to third in the pecking order it was as ironic as buses – New Zealand had waited a decade for a world-class hooker to come along and then three arrived at once. Despite seemingly having been pushed to the outer, Reid never stopped giving of his best and he never stopped trying to

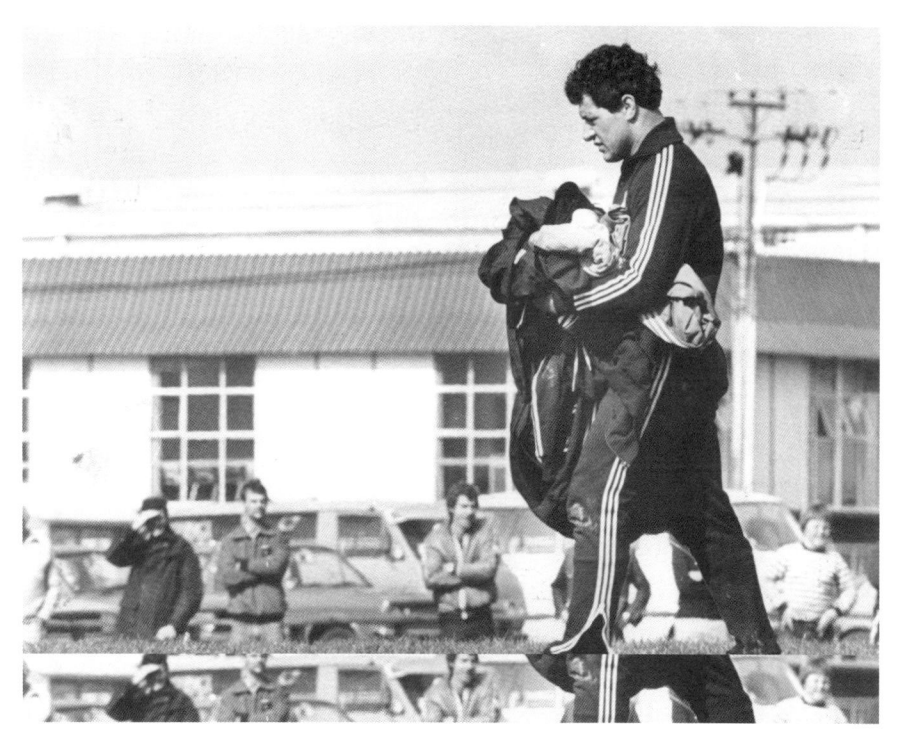

Hika Reid finds himself on housekeeping duty for the All Blacks in 1982. *New Zealand Herald*

add to his tally of test caps. He never lost his confidence and continued to believe the recall would one day come. That was Reid – positive, positive, positive. A believer that he could succeed as long as he applied himself. He was about to find out whether that theory would hold true regardless of how tough the task was.

'When I got to Hamilton and met the doctors there, I was told I had leukaemia. It was then that it all hit me. That explained why I had been feeling fatigued and why my spleen had been enlarged. I had just thought it was the old war wounds playing up.

'I can remember, though, I still thought I would be able to head out to Fiji with the Maori team. I said I couldn't really start any treatment until I came back.

'But the specialist told me that a normal level for white blood cells was 4.5 to nine. The danger area is 0.5 and that is when they start to get quite concerned. My level was 0.17. She told me that I was lucky to still be standing and that I could be in real trouble if I caught the flu or had a dodgy curry or something. Now that was poignant as whenever we went away with the Maori team, the first thing all the coaches and managers would do was find a good place to have a curry.

'I can remember after getting the initial news I then had to go off to see this young doctor and he had to test my bone marrow to see how far the cancer had spread. I said to him, "What's the verdict, doc?" It was Hairy Cell, a very aggressive and very rare strain and it was throughout my body. I thought shit, it's all over. I could envisage myself being very sick and dying. I was scheduled to go and see another specialist in the afternoon but again I thought stuff this, I'm going for a run. As I was running, I thought about how I was going to break the news to my wife. I started to think about all the things around the house I hadn't done. The house was a mess. I had started some work in the bathroom and hadn't finished it. I was thinking about my poor wife and all the things I hadn't done with my kids.'

In the space of an hour, Reid's dreams had been smashed. The short term was in turmoil. There would be no trip to Fiji. He wouldn't be at Waikato Stadium either. Longer term he couldn't see himself at the helm of the Steamers. That was his dream. At 47 he had developed significant coaching experience, having had stints with Harlequins, London Irish and Blackheath in the UK. He loved his job developing talent in the Bay of Plenty and coaching coaches but he always imagined there were other things on the horizon. He wanted a job in the bigtime. The Bay would be his first choice but any NPC team would do. And from there who knows where his career could take him.

But once the news of his leukaemia was delivered, he couldn't even be sure he would be at the helm of his family for Christmas. He was conscious that no one had been talking in time limits. No one had given any indication of how long he had left. He felt for sure, however, that he would be looking at weeks, maybe months if he were lucky.

The tragedy would be overwhelming. This was Hika Reid, the man who stormed all over the Cardiff Arms Park in 1980 and scored one of the finest tries that famous old ground had ever seen. He was the original modern hooker – rugged enough to operate efficiently at the coalface but athletic enough to canter in the wide spaces. He was clutched close to the heart of not only New Zealanders but many in the UK too. His immortality was assured when legendary Scottish commentator Bill McLaren referred to him as "Hika the hooker from Ngongotaha" as he called that breathtaking try.

Reid epitomised all that was good about All Black rugby. He was strong, fit, talented and skilful. The thought of him being taken early sent shock waves through the rugby community. The family rallied. The Bay dedicated their performance against the Lions to Reid. He was in the thoughts of the Maori team, too. And the thoughts of literally thousands of New Zealanders, and indeed Lions fans, too, were with him when they read about his diagnosis.

Reid had so many people willing him to turf out his unwelcome resident. No one wanted to see such a fine player, such a fine person, be denied a proper chance at the crease. The thing with cancer, though, is that it ultimately boils down to the motivation and dedication of the sufferer. Reid had immediately thought about death. He couldn't see that he had much hope. That was until he became armed with the full facts of what he was facing.

'I went to see the specialist in the afternoon and that changed everything. He told me the cancer was beatable. He said that normal people were only able to take so much chemotherapy and radiotherapy but that he was going to hit me seven days a week, 24 hours a day. He said that 80 per cent of people recover after their first dose of chemo. And for those who don't, they increase the dose. He gave me the window of hope that I needed. I knew there was a chance that I could beat it if I stayed positive and kept myself fit.'

Reid knew a thing or two about the importance of keeping fit. As a 19-year-old he had joined the Territorial Army with the sole purpose of putting his body through a torturous training regime. He was a talented rugby player but by his own admission he was as lazy as a butcher's dog. If he wanted to fulfil his unquestionable potential he needed to find more intensity and put himself around a bit more. When he rocked up to the

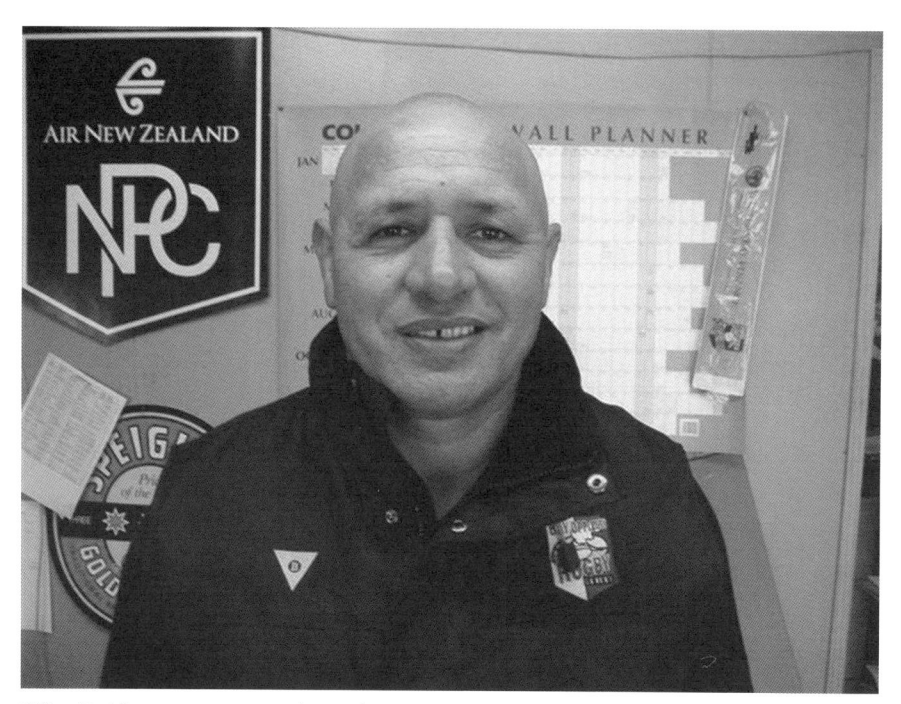

Hika Reid returns to work at the Bay of Plenty Rugby Union offices in 2005. *Bay of Plenty Rugby Union*

recruitment officer, Reid said he wanted to serve in the division that would expose him to the most brutal hard work. So he was sent away with the infantry as a rifleman. It was the hardest training he had ever done. He spent six weeks running and running and running. It made him realise how much the human body could endure.

By the end of his stint he was leaner and fitter than he had ever been. When he returned to the rugby field he fulfilled his goal of playing Senior A club rugby and more. By the end of the season he was in the Bay of Plenty NPC team. Three years later and he was an All Black.

He knew that his elevation to test honours had come about due to his dedication at training. His belief that the body had to be fit for the mind to operate at its most efficient stayed with him. So he knew the instant he was diagnosed that his mind and body would need to operate in tandem to defeat the leukaemia. And he knew for them to be at their most effective, they had to be in their best condition.

His chemotherapy was taken between boxing sessions, weight sessions and cycle sessions. When he wasn't in his room he was walking the corridors. He worked out that a circuit of the hospital was about 250 metres. He kept pounding the corridors, getting the miles under his belt. The fitter he was the more likely he was to repel the invaders who were attacking his white blood cells before they could form.

'A friend of mine rang from England and she reminded me to always remain positive. I was drinking gallons of water as I had been encouraged to do that to help flush out all the waste that is created when you undergo chemo. I was learning Maori at the time and every time I went to pee I chanted, "Get out of my body you pest, get out of me now." I was being observed at 3 am and 5 am. I was up at those times so I would do something on my Swiss ball, maybe some weights or ride on the bike. I was also doing some boxing at the time and I was imagining that I was the young white blood cells attacking the cancer. That's the type of thought process I had.

'Whenever I had visitors I always made sure I was dressed and up. I didn't want anyone to see me looking sickly and lying in bed. I always had to put my mask on. The chemo not only kills the bad cells, it also kills the good cells and you are very depleted of energy. I needed to be fit so I could rebuild my energy and feel I was rejuvenating the good healthy cells.'

There were several factors driving Reid. He knew he desperately wanted to live. Prior to his diagnosis he had burned with ambition for his coaching career. He was passionate about his work in the Bay and by all accounts good at it too. Like all ambitious people he wanted to progress. His eye was always roaming for potential opportunities.

But as he lay in hospital with the chemo draining into him, his perspective shifted. His career faded slightly in importance. He wanted to elevate his family higher up his list of priorities. The thought of leaving his family behind was terrifying. He definitely wasn't ready for that. He needed more time with them. Time to go on holiday and to help with homework. Just time to be a dad and enjoy the experience. And besides, he felt his dedication to work – as well as an overexposure to radiation through the numerous X-rays he endured throughout his playing career – had been the cause of his leukaemia in the first place. He was being stretched too far by his various demands and he was stressed. Rugby would no longer account for 80 per cent of his life.

It wasn't just family that became more important. The planned visit by his friends from the UK took on huge significance. Joining them in Christchurch for the first Lions versus All Blacks test was a major goal. Reid would envisage himself with his friends and those positive thoughts gave him added motivation. He would be out of hospital in time for the 25 June encounter. That would be significant. It would be the first major victory against the disease. The plan was he would endure one week intensive chemotherapy, then his body would kick in and continue the recovery so that by the end of three weeks he would be in a position to persuade the doctors he was winning the war.

Unfortunately that meant he wouldn't be able to take his place at a packed stadium at Rotorua on a glorious winter evening. At least, though, the Bay provided the perfect distraction and mental boost by delivering a classic underdog performance. Sure they lost, but the province was euphoric. The Lions had come to town claiming to be the best-prepared side ever. The Steamers rattled them and had every right to claim a moral victory.

The following week, Reid's spirits were lifted further. The Maori were playing the Lions only a few hundred metres from his hospital room. He wasn't distraught that he wasn't there. He had accepted that to achieve his goal of being in Christchurch for the first test, the Maori game was one he would have to watch on TV. As much as it hurt not to be in the coaches' box and have an active role as the drama unfolded, the Maori game was going to be a casualty of his leukaemia.

'The hospital didn't have SKY so I had to wait for it to come on normal TV. I could hear the crowd coming in through the window and I had a feeling that something good was going on for us. I had to switch off my mobile phone as Matt Te Pou [Maori coach] was ringing me after the game, but I didn't want to know the score. I wanted to watch the game on TV without knowing who had won. It was brilliant.'

It was just the fillip he needed to further boost his spirits and keep his recovery on track. When his chemo finished Reid was in good physical and mental shape. The hours he had spent on his bike and Swiss ball had enabled him to respond well to his treatment. The war he had waged had been effective. He had refused to allow the leukaemia any opportunity to attack his white blood cells. Not only was his body strong, his mind had been strong, too, continually sending out the orders to all corners of his body that the invaders were to be repelled. Once again, Reid had shown that dedication to a tough physical regime could help him achieve his goals.

He had been in the 80 per cent grouping the doctors had talked about and as a result Reid's medical team were happy for him to take off to the South Island and enjoy his long-planned trip. They were amazed at the speed of his recovery. He wasn't celebrating, though. His white blood cell count had lifted enough to show he was responding to the treatment. But even as this book went to print, it was still on the low side. He still has bronchitis as a consequence of his immune system being way less effective and he is conscious of having to watch his diet. He's more on the edge of the woods rather than out of them entirely.

But the determination that got him through the worst part of his ordeal is still very much with him. He was at work pretty much as soon as he got back from his Lions venture. And he returned in typical Reid fashion. 'He came back unannounced,' says Bay of Plenty chief executive Paul Abbot. 'He wandered into the office and pretty much said, "I'm back, what do you want me to do?" We were delighted to see him. It had been a real shock for everyone in the Bay to learn about Hika's leukaemia.

'He is one of life's characters and one of the few guys with the mana to walk into any rugby club in the Bay and get people to respond. He had wanted to keep his diagnosis and treatment as secret as he could. He didn't want people to see him ill and he certainly didn't want to make a song and dance about it. We never knew whether he would be able to come back, or in what capacity he would be able to return. We always hoped he would be able to, but we just didn't know.

'He's had to slow down a bit. Standing out on those cold winter nights coaching club sides took it out of him a bit. But he still goes above and beyond the call of duty for the province. He's got so much rugby experience that if he feels it is the right thing for him to do, we would see him as one of the leading contenders to coach the NPC team should that job become available.'

The fact that Reid has reduced his commitments – he's dropped off his work with the Maori and stepped aside from coaching the Bay of Plenty development team – should not be seen as a dilution of his ambition. He's had to tailor his workload to his physical limits. He focuses more now on his role as a development officer and he will play a key role for the Steamers NPC team in 2006, advising on a number of issues.

Sure, his family take up more of his time now, as do those chores around the house that he never got round to doing, but his coaching career means a lot to him and he wants to be successful. His primary aim, though, is far more basic. 'Just to survive another year would be a good achievement. You always have these doubts that it is going to kick in again. I can't afford to be complacent. I think what I learned when I was in the hospital is how fragile life is. I can remember seeing an old fella in the oncology ward when I was wandering around. A few days later and he wasn't there any more.

'I got a lot of good support from friends and family that saw me through. Andy Haden [former All Black] was a great comfort to me. His brother Richard had the same cancer as I had and he has been in remission for 10 years. Andy said if you put all the cancers in a jar, ours would be one of the best ones to have. That wasn't to lessen what I was going through, it was to help me.

'So I think I have learned not to worry so much about the things I can't control. That's both in life and with my coaching. I used to get really frustrated with little things. They would get on top of me. Now I can see they don't really matter so much. I have got to be in control of my blood pressure and remind myself every now and again that I have been given a second chance. I'm much more relaxed now, except when I'm driving. Man, some people frustrate me when I'm driving. They don't have the vision. They can't read the play.'

It wouldn't be a surprise if Reid, in time, offered to help out those drivers who struggle for form on the road. Helping others is a big part of the man. There could be no better endorsement of his humanity and compassion than the way he handled his diagnosis and subsequent treatment. When word leaked out he had leukaemia, a number of media outlets requested interviews to tell his story. He refused. He didn't want to be in the spotlight at such an uncertain time. But now that he is more in control and aware that he could be an inspiration to others, he'll talk to anyone if they reckon it might help.

When the words are coming out of the mouth of Hika Reid, it's a safe bet they will be helping those who hear them.

Hika Reid played seven tests and 31 games for the All Blacks, scoring six tries. He also played 85 times for the Bay of Plenty, 25 for Wellington and regularly featured at hooker for the New Zealand Maori team. He was also the winner on two occasions of the Tom French Cup – the annual award for the most outstanding Maori player. When he finished playing he enjoyed professional coaching stints at the Harlequins club, London Irish and then Blackheath. He returned to New Zealand in 2003 to take up a role as a development officer with the Bay of Plenty Rugby Union and was also used by the New Zealand Maori team in 2005 as a technical adviser.

11

EAMONN DOYLE

New Zealand National Indoor Rowing Champion 2002

Eamonn Doyle really had no right to be at the world indoor rowing championships in February 2005. It wasn't that he didn't deserve his place in an elite field – a field that contained a handful of Olympians. He most certainly did. He proved that when he finished 27th out of 80 competitors. It's just that he really had no right to be alive. No one does when they drive a motorcycle at 143 km/h into a power pole and are then catapulted into a wall.

Even those with only a rudimentary grasp of physics can hazard a reasonable guess that the human form comes off second best when propelled into a stationary structure at that sort of velocity.

Doyle was definitely runner-up in his particular collision. Perhaps it was fortunate he was plunged into a coma for the four weeks after his accident. That way he didn't have to hear the doctors at Auckland's Mercy Hospital tell his parents the prognosis. Death was the most likely outcome. Probably the only outcome. But there was just a sliver of hope that he may somehow regain consciousness and live with major brain-damage and paralysis.

Neither of Doyle's parents, Erin and William, could think about either scenario. Certainly the second option was preferable. A devoted and loving mother, Erin Doyle wanted her boy back. In any shape or form, it didn't matter.

But the medics couldn't see how it was going to happen. The injuries Doyle had incurred were severe. His whole face had been smashed, which was why his head was swollen to almost twice its natural size. The doctors were making an educated assumption that there would be significant brain damage. Doyle's right knee-cap had been virtually torn off and there were broken ribs. There was severe bruising everywhere and no accurate way of telling whether the spine had been permanently damaged.

If the doctors had been forced to assess Doyle's chances of living in percentage terms, they would have said somewhere between zero and 10 per cent. It wasn't looking good. Things never do when you are on a life support machine, unable to breathe or conduct any of the functions necessary to exist.

A couple of weeks after being brought in, Doyle's chances, already tenuous, slipped to infinitesimal. He was suffering from pneumonia, a potential killer of the fit and healthy, an almost certain killer of the seriously ill. The family priest was summoned to read the last rites. For Doyle's parents the last vestiges of hope were all but gone. Their son, only 19, was slipping away. There appeared no way back. No one at Mercy Hospital could offer any hope. All the Doyles could do was pray. Hope that their faith would be rewarded with a miracle. Their son's body had endured too much trauma. Medical science is only capable of so much. Sometimes there are no answers. Sometimes the damage is too severe.

No matter how many times they asked God to intervene, they knew that, really, it was down to Eamonn to somehow fight for his life. They knew it was down to him to somehow find the will to live. And as much as they loved their son, they just couldn't be sure there was a fire burning deep inside his belly.

Doyle was one of life's cruisers. A teenager perennially stuck in neutral. He had meandered his way through his time at St Peter's College in Auckland and had left with no real plan for his future. There were always ideas but he wasn't keeping the sort of company that would win approving nods at afternoon tea with his parents. His exposure to less savoury characters was perhaps preventing him from ever getting ahead. He knew he was flirting with danger, but didn't care enough to actively put his life on a track more likely to collide with good fortune.

As a result, when he woke late on the morning of 12 April 2000, he suffered a collision all right, but it was one utterly devoid of good fortune.

As Doyle remembers it: 'I was labouring on construction sites round the place. I had no real direction. I hadn't put any real thought into anything. I was just floating.

'I was working at a site in Parnell at the end of the Domain. I was supposed to be there at six in the morning. I had been working for a new guy for about a week. He was a really choice boss. I really liked him. He was just real particular about being punctual.

'I didn't want to mess up because I was enjoying the job. I had been out the night before, getting on it. I came home around three, had a few hours' sleep and woke about 6.45 am. I freaked out because I was supposed to be there three-quarters of an hour ago.

'I thought a couple of hours' sleep would do it. It was obviously a major error of judgement. I jumped on my bike and because I was so late and in a bit of rush and there was no traffic around at that time of the morning, I was riding quite fast. I thrashed the bike wherever I went. It was a 1994 Japanese sports bike so it had a lot of power.

'I was still a bit drunk and a little bit tired. I wiped out on Mountain Road. I came round a long right-hander and my bike hit a power pole and ripped it clean out of the ground. I came off the bike and flew into the air, straight into a wall. That was what stopped me. The speedometer was stuck at 143 km/h. People say I can't have been going that fast. I am not proud to say it. It's a bit embarrassing. But I was drunk and drunk 19-year-olds don't make the best decisions.

'There were a couple of people out walking their dogs. Apparently after I crashed I tried to get up and get my bike off the road. And then I collapsed. I have got no recollection of what happened. None at all. I woke up four and a half weeks later.'

No medics can say why Doyle woke up. In their business, there are

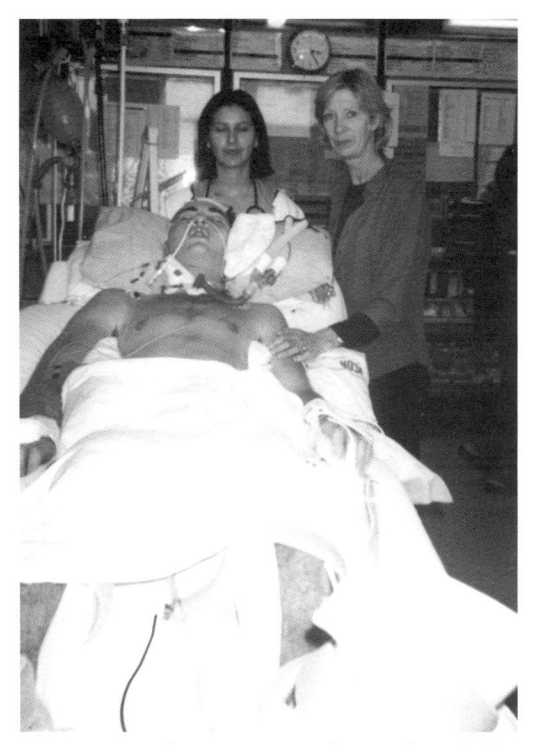

Eamonn Doyle recovers in hospital with his mother, Erin (right) looking on.

occasional miracles. Amid all the suffering and death, there can, every now and again, be an unexplained moment of joy. Doyle himself is under no illusions as to what saved him. As a devout Catholic, he believes he survived thanks to the grace of God. He can't offer any other explanation. His family were overjoyed. Their boy was back. Yet, there was an irony looming that none of the Doyles knew – opening his eyes was the beginning, not the end of Eamonn's nightmare.

It was only now that he had regained consciousness that the doctors could fully assess the extent of the damage. Amazingly, it was not as bad as it should have been. There wasn't any serious skeletal damage. There was widespread bruising. His lower back in particular was a problem. His right knee-cap had been smashed and there was a minor problem with his right hand.

Given the speed he was travelling when he hit the power pole, he had no right to get off so lightly. But there was one serious problem – his brain had suffered a major trauma. He was in possession of his basic faculties. He could speak, he knew who he was and he seemed pretty with it. There was no Hollywood major amnesia. Trouble had been stored for later, though.

Jim Noble, who was assigned as Doyle's physiotherapist, paints a picture of how Doyle's brain had effectively endured its own distinct experience during the crash.

'The severity of the injury to his brain and the location were the two most hazardous features. He had a very rough time in the hospital and they had to decompress his brain in the X-ray department because his pressure shot up substantially.

'He came very close to not surviving at all. When he came off his motorbike he must have gone over the handlebars coming round to the left. He was travelling head first but backwards towards the wall. He struck the wall on the top right of his head, above his right ear. When he hit the wall, his brain headed towards that first point of impact. It compressed the skull on that point and it tore away structures on the other side of the brain.

'Then it came to a halt and the reverse happened so the brain sloshed back in the direction it came. It produced a double feature. That trauma ripped some blood vessels that started to bleed with a vengeance. In his case, because he got hit so close to the hospital, he was there in a very short space of time.

'Initially when they got him there, they took a chunk off his skull and evacuated the bleeding. They had to open up the lining of his brain. He was sent back to the ward. But a few hours later he was due to go back to the X-ray department to get another set of films. On the way there the pressure shot up dramatically. They didn't have time to take him to theatre. The house surgeon who was at his side had to whip a piece of skull off and hurriedly decompress the brain.

'The surgery report said they were all showered with blood as a result of the pressure. If that had not been dealt with promptly Eamonn would have died right there on the spot.'

There were times, many times in fact, when Doyle wished that he had just died there on the spot. He had been reduced, albeit temporarily, to not even a shadow of his former self. He was struggling to walk. He was in constant pain and his brain was having difficulty coping with the most basic functions. He was being driven by a brain that only had enough power to drive a five-year-old.

Slowly, ever so slowly, his functions would recover. But it was a painstaking process and not one Doyle always had the necessary willpower to find a way through.

'It is the weirdest thing, having that gap in your life. It takes a long time to get your head round that you have been in a coma. A few people ask me what it is like. It is just like going to sleep and waking up. I had no idea. When I woke up I wanted to go and ride my bike until my mate said, "No, no, you crashed your bike." I didn't believe him. I didn't even know I had been in a coma.

'I was bedridden for weeks. Being laid up for a couple of months without moving – I had to learn how to balance again. While I was in a coma they didn't know whether I was going to be paralysed. At the darkest hour they told my mum they didn't think I would survive and if I did, the best they could hope for was that I would be a vegetable.

'I went to a rehab centre for a few months. It took a while, probably four or five months before I could walk unaided. I was really weak. I felt like I was never going to get my body back. I kept saying to my mum, "Am I going to feel this wasted for the rest of my life?" My handwriting was like a scribble. There was so much to work on. It was like being a toddler again. It was like I was starting my life again. I wasn't able to do much. My arm was still smashed and in a sling. I could walk maybe 100 metres.

'They were the darkest times. I was really scared. In the infancy of my recovery I really wished I hadn't pulled through. I was totally wasted. I lost 20 kg. I was finding my life pretty hard. I thought, stuff this, and I wished I hadn't pulled through. I couldn't see how I was going to get better. I thought this can't be me for the rest of my life.'

He found life at the rehabilitation centre unbelievably depressing. Being tasked every day with simple activities that he felt were beneath him. The horrid thing for Doyle was that many of the activities were beyond him. But due to the nature of his brain injury he was unaware, or maybe just in denial about his reduced physical and mental capacity.

It was at the rehabilitation centre that Doyle met Noble. The immediate impression formed by Noble was that Doyle was going to struggle to regain normality.

'When I first saw Eamonn, he came to the workshop for a look. At that time he said he wanted to fix up a motorbike. So we acquired an old banger of a thing and I asked him to dismantle it. I remember quite distinctly he took the front wheel off and there was an axle pin and a washer when the wheel was taken out. He threw them in the bucket and I suggested it would be a good idea if he put them together so the bits didn't get lost. He took a look in the bucket and said it didn't matter because they wouldn't all fit together. At that stage he had a very poor awareness of how things operated.

'I didn't form a great impression of his long-term prospects. Some people lose the ability to sense when things are square or upright. He continued on for a period of time, drifting, not being able to do very much at all. He was insulted at having to come to the rehabilitation centre because there were all these sick and disabled people and he didn't recognise himself as one. He didn't think there was anything wrong with him at all. He almost lacked completely self-awareness.

'It was a severe disability because anyone who has a problem and doesn't think they have, really has got a big problem.'

By the time Doyle was allowed back home to live, he was mired in a deep depression. He was being plagued by thoughts of suicide. All he wanted to do was sit in his bedroom, flick the lights off and hope the time would pass. But he couldn't get the clock to tick any quicker. He couldn't stop the nightmares. He couldn't recover his confidence and nor could he lose the lingering regret.

Doyle wasn't besieged by self-pity. He knew his predicament was his own fault. He had been the master of his own fate. But still, it didn't make things any easier.

'I hated it. It was dark times. For a long time I didn't want to leave the house. I didn't even want to leave my room. I was so fragile and unsure of everything. I was so confused and bewildered about everything. I was just hanging in there.

'These were my prime years. It was really difficult to accept I missed out being 19, 20, 21, 22. Knowing all my mates were out there living it up and having a good time. It's not easy.'

Noble could see that Doyle needed some direction in his life. He needed some routine and structure to help him forge a way out of the darkness. Almost 18 months after returning home, Doyle had made significant physical progress. He was living a reasonably normal life in the sense that he could function well enough to enjoy the trappings of youth.

He needed to be in better shape psychologically, though, to drive home the final yards of the physical recovery. Doyle was still living in his shell. He was still tentative, directionless and lacking confidence and motivation. Noble wanted to create focus, offer a more positive diversion. It came when Doyle expressed an interest in rowing as part of his physical rehabilitation.

'Eamonn mentioned that he had done some rowing before his injury. I picked on that because that activity involves a routine. I utilised that as a hook on which to hang all my other interventions with him.

'So I set up a routine where he had to come initially once a day and then twice a day to train. That, in Eamonn's case, was very helpful. For all the other things that were going wrong in his life, at least he had this basic routine to fall back on. His lack of awareness and inability to plan meant he could be quite irrational at times. In terms of his physical capacity he was starting to make progress but it was very, very hard work.'

It was Noble's belief that it was harder work than it should have been because Doyle was not necessarily living his life on the straight and narrow. Doyle certainly wasn't squeaky clean and Noble felt there were elements of Doyle's private life that were hindering his progress. He wanted Doyle to clean up his act and made that clear in terms that could never be described as ambiguous.

It was rowing, and that ultimatum from Noble, that provided the catalyst for Doyle to turn his life around. He'd done some rowing at St Peter's. Only a little but enough to know he enjoyed it. It was easy to see why. He stands at 2.03 metres and has the perfect physique for the sport.

When he first rekindled his interest he could only manage five or six minutes before he would collapse. As he gradually built his stamina, Noble would up the length of time Doyle spent on the machine. Doyle briefly joined a crew on the water, but the early morning requirements were too much for his body to deal with.

His participation would be confined to indoor work, an increasingly popular and competitive offshoot of the sport.

'From starting off only being able to do five minutes, it was a case of building up week by week. The main thing was it made me feel a lot better. It cleared my mind so I decided it was a good thing to stick at.'

Indeed it was a good thing to stick at. By 2002 Doyle was not only showing signs of being a seriously good rower, he was becoming a better person too. The nightmares were easing off. The depression was being kept at bay. His accident was no longer a catastrophe devoid of any redeeming feature. He was going to the well of despair and drawing black memories only to convert them into the most productive fuel.

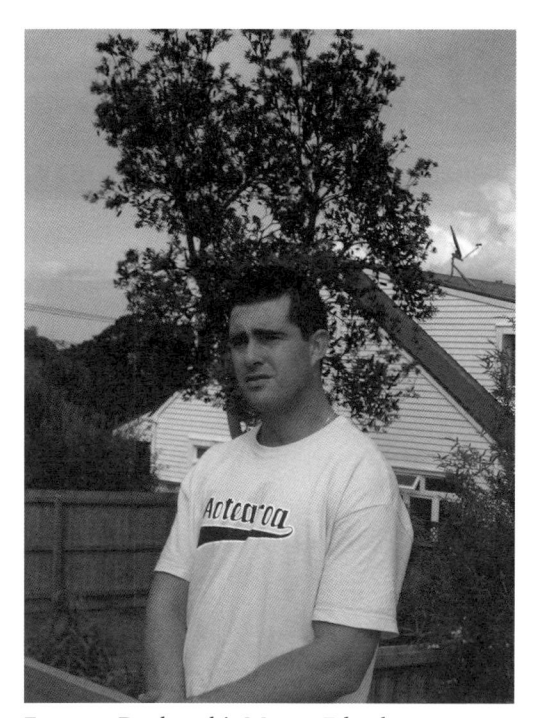

Eamonn Doyle at his Mount Eden home.

Rowing appeared to be his long-lost calling. It appeared to be the very reason God had plucked him from death's door. He was no longer a drifter operating without clear goals. The rebel was no longer without a cause. He had some ambition and Noble could see the transition.

'I had used a video during some of my original discussions with Eamonn. His physical appearance was what you would expect of a young guy doing nothing very much at all. He was quite slack and had long hair and all the rest of it. In his case, his posture gave away his basic attitude to life, which was there was no point in trying because everything goes wrong anyway. He was just waiting for something to come and knock him over because everything always had in the past. He slumped. He never sat upright.

'That gradually changed when he got fitter. The approach was to pick a level of training where he could see he was succeeding with a level of effort. He could see if he did this much training he would be able to get to that kind of mark.

'It gradually came to be appreciated by him that there was a predictable element in life and that not everything was random. Flicking the coin, he generally expected it to come down the wrong way round.'

Doyle took a massive step towards realising he was in control of his own destiny in October 2002. His performance reached a point where Noble entered him in the New Zealand indoor championships.

Stamina was still an issue, but over 500 metres Doyle had the size, physique and determination to compete with the very best. A top quality field assembled in the gym at Epsom Girls Grammar School in Auckland. It was the first time Doyle had competed seriously at anything. He was understandably nervous and as a consequence ripped into the machine with no strategy other than to empty his tank. He did exactly that and one minute 21 seconds later, he was crowned the winner.

'I was ecstatic. I hadn't felt that good in a long time. I can still remember that day now. It restored my pride, my self-esteem. I was surprised. I didn't know I had it in me. I went flat tack. They've got a big screen showing where your boat is. I didn't even look at it. I just went flat out.'

Later that day his mother took him down to Newmarket for a celebratory feed. She can remember sitting in the car watching Eamonn walk up the street. 'I saw this giant. I saw this boy floating on air. It was something I never thought I would see.'

A few months later and he was on the winner's podium again after winning the Auckland Inter-Gym event. This time he was racing over 1 km and only just managed to hold on after heading out too fast.

It was enough for Noble to mention the World Championships in Boston. If it was far-fetched, a tad preposterous even, Doyle didn't take the time to think about it. The boy who had been a whisker away from death and saved by the quick thinking of a hospital house surgeon, was a boy on a mission. At least he was once Noble delivered his ultimatum.

Doyle had huge potential. He could really make a name for himself at this rowing lark. He could one day make the switch to an outdoor crew, go to the Olympics or World Championships. These possibilities were real.

Which is why Noble threatened to withdraw his help unless Doyle committed himself entirely to the training programme. 'When we were talking I put the acid on him. I said, "If you are going to do it, you have got to do it properly." That made a big difference. He really trained very hard. It was brutal.

'That talk really helped him turn the corner when he was preparing to go to the World Championships. Once he started the preparation for that, then his physical capacity started to improve a great deal.'

It was nine months of hell for Doyle. But a very different hell to the one he had endured in the first three years after his accident. This was a self-inflicted hell that carried enormous physical and mental benefits. The training regime was extraordinarily tough. Twice a day, six days a week he'd be in the gym. More experienced athletes than Doyle have been broken by such excessive demands.

Maybe, though, Doyle had more life experience driving him than other athletes. He was here only by the grace of God and Doyle knew he owed a debt. To repay it, he had to deliver. Success had eluded him before his accident. He had survived for a reason.

'Before I went to Boston I went to the performance lab over at the Shore. They run a whole lot of tests on you to see what your flexibility is like and all these other tests. After that they draw up a training programme. I was following that regime for nine months. That was hard. At the end of it I have never been in such good condition. I was in mean shape.

'I'll just forever be amazed. I was being given a second chance. I wanted to make good use of this opportunity. That was the inspiration for me. That was the driving force behind it. I would be thanking God, I suppose. I kept thinking how lucky I was. I mean 143 km/h ... you don't crash a bike at that speed and come away with your arms and your legs and your intellect intact. It doesn't happen.'

And you certainly don't end up making it into the world championships of a global sport. By the time Doyle left for Boston in February 2005, he was in quite spectacular physical condition. Strangers would have taken some major convincing this was a guy who had been in pieces four-and-a-half years earlier. But even though he was in prime physical shape, some of the psychological issues were still haunting Doyle.

Travelling long-haul for the first time nearly got the better of him. And existing away from home, never mind competing away from home, was a major ordeal. As a consequence he took his place in Boston's elite field – there were outdoor Olympians such as New Zealand's George Bridgewater – not quite in the frame of mind he would have liked. There was also a huge amount of background noise that Doyle found hard to concentrate through.

In the end he finished his 2 km race about 10 seconds slower than he was capable of. It was still enough to finish 27th out of 80 entrants. Not bad for an elite rower with years of experience. An incredible achievement for someone who only took up the sport three years earlier as a consequence of suffering a horrendous accident that almost killed him.

As someone who had seen Doyle at his lowest physical and mental ebbs, Noble knew this was huge. A staggering accomplishment when he sits back and recalls the battered, depressed young man he first met in 2000.

'To be able to handle that amount of training was a very big accomplishment. The hassles he had to deal with and the nature of his injury make it a monumental achievement really. I was greatly impressed with him.

'I would think he is inspirational. The race that he was in was the last race of the day. He would have done quite a lot better if there were some means of him avoiding the noise. The guys next to him were screaming their lungs out and he is easily distracted. I think he would have knocked 10 seconds off his time.'

For Doyle, it was so much more than just a great achievement in a rowing race. It was the final proof he had turned his life around and laid the ghosts of his past to rest. The troubled teenager effectively died on the morning of 12 April 2000. What emerged in the shell of Doyle's body was a more complete young man – someone with drive, purpose and ambition. The old Doyle would never have made it to Boston. He simply wouldn't have had the inclination or patience.

The new Doyle was a much-improved model. There was intrinsic motivation now. He was driven by the knowledge he was so very fortunate to be given a second chance. He was driven by the need to succeed and make the pain and suffering all worth while. And who could say he didn't do all that and more? It's a sign of his newfound self-confidence and hunger to prove himself that there is just the faintest hint of disappointment that he didn't quite nail his best effort in Boston.

'I had never travelled before. I was jet-lagged. The nerves were so bad for about three nights, including the day before the race, I was up until 5.30 am. I couldn't stop thinking about it. I had very little sleep so I was a bit of a mess on the day of the race. But I gave it my all and I was stoked. It was a massive achievement. I was competing for everyone. We were celebrating what we had all come through together. I don't know how to explain those feelings but I did think it was a bit ridiculous that I was in Boston competing at that level.

'My rowing has been paramount. I don't know where I would be without my rowing or Jim Noble. He saved my life, he really did. I'm a totally different guy. I think I'm more motivated. Before my accident I was getting into a bit of trouble. Hanging out with people I shouldn't have been hanging out with. I wasn't really too sure which way I was going. I was up to no good. I didn't care. I'm a reformed character now.

'Good things have come of my accident. I don't know what I would be like if it had not been for this life-changing event. I am not forgetting how lucky I am.'

Luck and the grace of God took him so far. But Eamonn Doyle did the rest.

Eamonn Doyle was crowned New Zealand Indoor Rowing Champion in October 2002. In June 2003 he won the Auckland Inter-Gym event. In February 2005 he finished 27th out of 80 competitors at the World Indoor Rowing Championship. He is currently being encouraged and mentored by former Olympic champion rower and current America's Cup team member, Rob Waddell. While a switch to outdoor rowing is a possibility further down the line, Doyle is currently pouring all his energy into trying to win a place as a crew member on Team New Zealand's America's Cup 2007 challenge.

12

STEVE GURNEY

Coast to Coast Winner 1990, 1991, 1997-2003

The tear made tiny ripples when it slid off Steve Gurney's cheek and fell into the Waimakariri River. It had been shed in jubilation but inspired by grief. It marked the passing of the last two years. They had been two years during which Gurney had suffered a physical and mental torment more intense than anything he had ever encountered as an elite endurance athlete.

As he sat in his kayak, he tried to take it all in. His mind flooded with memories he would rather forget. He had a vision of being pinned down by a roomful of doctors who were trying to sedate him in Malaysia. He recalled the drama of being squeezed into a tiny Lear Jet, his life support machine in tow, as he flew to the hospital in Singapore that would perform miracles to keep him alive. He remembered getting back to Christchurch, almost 30 kg lighter and so weak he could hardly stand up.

He exorcised those demons, dipped his paddle back in the water and continued on his way. He was far enough ahead of the rest of the field to know that he was going to win his third Coast to Coast title – the race most endurance athletes consider the benchmark for multi-sport adventures. He'd won the Coast to Coast twice before, but he knew as he made his way through the Waimakariri Gorge in 1997, that this particular victory would forever hold a special place in his heart.

Hard Men Fight Back

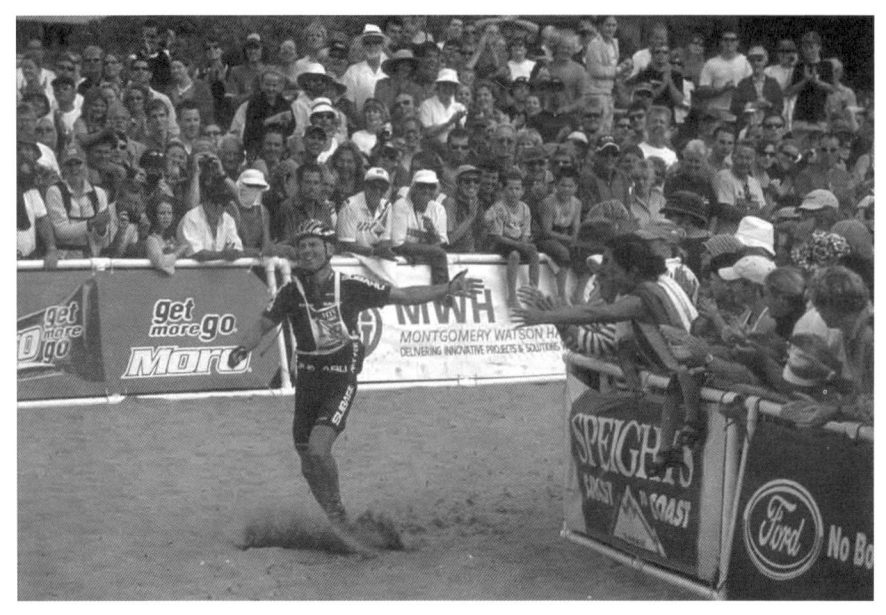

Steve Gurney high-fives the crowd on his way to his fifth successive Coast to Coast title in 2001.

When Gurney finally reached Sumner beach in Christchurch it signalled that his astonishing recovery was complete. As his chest went through the finishing tape he felt as if he was running into a new life on the other side. The elation swamped him. For the last two years he had feared that he had lost his sport forever. That thought had plunged him into a serious depression. Without being able to compete in multi-sport races around the world, he feared there would be a void in his life that he would never be able to fill. Those dark times had plagued him since November 1994, when he accepted an invitation to take part in an adventure race in Malaysia.

1994 had been a gruelling year for the then 31-year-old Gurney. He'd spent much of it competitively mountain biking in the United States. He was probably in need of some rest and recovery when he was offered a place in a five man team taking part in the Raid Gauloises – a seriously tough adventure through the jungles of Borneo. He probably should have declined. But saying no wasn't in Gurney's nature. He was a competitive beast and this type of race was exactly what floated his boat. Besides, there was some pretty serious prize money on offer. There would be time to rest once he got back to Christchurch. As it turned out, by the time he did eventually get back to Christchurch, he would barely be able to get enough of resting.

For a while, everything had been going exactly as planned in Borneo. Gurney and his team-mates had cut an impressive swathe through the jungle. They were travelling so much faster than the organisers had predicted that they were days rather than hours ahead of schedule.

On the final leg of their adventure they entered the Mulu caves. 'It is the biggest cave system in the world – there are still parts unexplored in there,' says Gurney. 'We just went through one piece that was three or four hours long. There are quite a few bats in the cave and these bats would crap all over the floor and there was a creek running through the cave. The water looked quite clean but it must have been contaminated with bat crap as well. I can't prove it but it looks like I caught leptospirosis that these bats were carrying. You get it from rodents and from cattle. You contract it by getting the faeces or the urine of a rodent in a scratch or cut or in your mouth. I had a cut on my shin. I didn't have long pants on and I didn't have the cut dressed so it probably got in through there. It is like a blood poisoning. It has a seven-day incubation period.'

Oblivious to the deadly infection he had contracted, Gurney trooped on with his team, winning the event by some margin. The organisers had been left embarrassed. They had been planning on things taking a little longer and the prizegiving had been set for the end of the week. Gurney and his team would have to hang around in the small town of Miri for another five days. No problem. They were all physically drained from their exertions and it wasn't such a bad spot to gently explore at their leisure. But a few days later, Gurney was beginning to discover that the bacterial time bomb inside him was ticking.

'About five days after winning the race I started feeling a bit crook. I had sore joints and a fever – it was a bit like flu symptoms. I thought that I was all right. We were due to fly home a few days after I started feeling really bad. I thought I would just see it out and wait to get back to New Zealand to see a doctor if the symptoms were still persisting. I had been pretty laid out for this race so I wasn't too worried. I was taking aspirin. We were in the hotel doing a couple of day trips and doing some sightseeing. I didn't feel well enough to do some of those things and even though it was stinking hot I ended up feeling so cold that I had to have hot baths.

'Just as I was starting to feel really bad I met this guy at the hotel who was an expat Kiwi and he advised me that I should ring a doctor. So I did and the doctor said, "That sounds really bad – you need to get to hospital." All the planes were really full because there were a lot of people attending the prizegiving. So we ended up waiting until after the prizegiving and by then I was pretty bad. I can't remember much of the plane flight.'

Fortunately for Gurney, his long-time friend John Howard was one of his team-mates. Howard had flown on an earlier flight out of Miri to Kuching, unaware of just how dramatically Gurney's health had deteriorated. Leptospirosis is a cussed and nasty bacterial infection. Gurney had been suffering from the first phase of the disease in Miri. He had the flu-like symptoms, the high fever, the chills, the severe headaches and the muscle aches. By the time he was airborne, he was moving into the second phase. His life was really in danger. He was jaundiced, his eyes had turned red and he had abdominal pain. He had become so delirious from the fever that the night before he had flown out he had been discovered trying to throw himself off the balcony of his hotel room.

That crazy behaviour had alerted Gurney's friends that he was not in a good way. Gurney was in much worse shape than anyone had previously thought, which is why Howard got a call shortly after he arrived in Kuching telling him to get back to the airport with an ambulance. Gurney landed a few hours later and was whisked to the nearest hospital. The longer the disease went untreated the greater the likelihood that Gurney would develop kidney damage, liver failure and respiratory distress. And if he developed those symptoms, the chances were pretty high that he would be flying back to Christchurch in a coffin.

'When I got to the airport it was pretty obvious Steve was very ill,' recalls Howard. 'We got him into the hospital at Kuching but that first night he was there he had a turn for the worse. They had to put him into intensive care as he had a circulatory collapse. Part of the problem was the doctors didn't really know what was wrong with him. They thought he might have had dengue fever but they couldn't be sure.

'Leptospirosis is very hard to diagnose. You need a blood culture to be sure so they were working on the premise that Steve might have had one of a number of things. It was a bit of an eye-opener for us because leptospirosis is actually quite easy to treat if you catch it early. It is quite common in that part of the world and a lot of athletes are exposed to it. A dose of antibiotics is normally enough to treat it in the early stages.'

The medics might not have been exactly sure what Gurney was suffering from, but they were positive he was in the advanced stage of whatever it was. The night after Gurney's circulatory system collapsed, Howard, who was in the room next door, heard his name being shouted by the doctors in his friend's room. They were trying to sedate Gurney. He was battling too hard to stay awake and fight the infection. The doctors were hoping to anaesthetise him and keep him in an induced coma to let his body focus on fighting the disease. But Gurney was lashing out – delirious and confused as to what was happening. The Malaysian doctors didn't have the combined strength to pin him down so Howard had to weigh in and restrain his old friend.

The nightmare was worsening. Howard knew how driven Gurney was. He knew that his friend would fight and fight and fight. He had never seen Gurney give up at anything he had ever tried. But this was maybe too much even for the super-fit, ultra-tenacious Gurney. His kidneys had stopped working and he was on dialysis. He couldn't breathe for himself and the doctors were still drawing blanks on what exactly they were up against.

'When Steve first arrived in Kuching,' says Howard, 'I remember he asked the doctor whether he was going to die. The doctor didn't say yes, but nor did he say no. He refused to say no and that hit home. I have to say, there was a time there when I thought Steve was going to die.

'After a few days in Kuching the doctors were becoming more discouraged. It was only a small medical facility and their resources had been really stretched. I think between the doctors and the medical

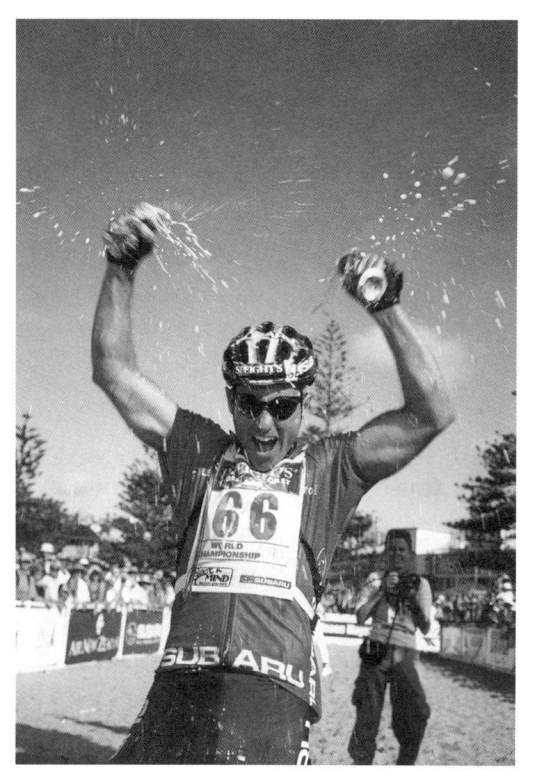

Steve Gurney celebrates winning the 1999 Coast to Coast. It was his third consecutive victory and fifth overall.

insurance people it was decided he should be moved to Singapore. The insurance company organised a flight on this tiny Lear Jet. We put him on the ambulance and then we had to get him on this plane, which was a real job. He had a machine breathing for him and we had to get him through this porthole that was only about a metre and a half wide. No one could carry him so I ended up having to do it. I had to manhandle him through the door while the others had to shove the machinery in that was breathing for him. It was so stressful and one of the most claustrophobic things I have ever done.

'We eventually got him on the plane and the pilot took off but then he started circling round the airport. After a while he decided the plane wasn't functioning properly so he landed. We had to get Steve off the plane, back on to the ambulance and then back into hospital. And all the time we were thinking that we would have to go through the whole ordeal again the next day.

'The next night they actually sent people over who had better equipment. They had a stretcher that wrapped around Steve's body and that made it much easier to carry him and get him on the plane. The flight only took about 25 to 30 minutes. But when we got to Singapore it just so happened there was a football match that night between Singapore and Malaysia. It meant the roads were really crowded and there were traffic jams. So getting Steve from the airport to the hospital took a bit longer than the doctors would have liked. Once we got him to the hospital he almost immediately started to improve. I don't think it was so much to do with the better medical facilities as the timing. All the antibiotics and treatment they had given him had started to make an impact by the time we got him there.'

It was a good job the antibiotics had started working as Gurney's lungs had filled with water before he left Kuching. His eyes had become what paint manufacturers would have described as outback red and his bones had started to protrude in places where once they had been concealed by well-toned flesh. By the time Gurney had regained consciousness and was out of danger, no one would ever have believed they were looking at one of the world's best multi-sport endurance athletes. He looked as if, rather than having just powered his way through the jungles of Borneo in record time, he had actually been lost in there for some time without much idea how to forage for himself. The idea of him being able to complete another gruelling Coast to Coast was laughable. He would be happy enough if he could just make it from one side of his hospital room to the other.

'They told me afterwards that they were a bit surprised I survived,' says Gurney. 'They thought I was too advanced. With these diseases, the earlier you get in the better, so now I take low-dose antibiotics before I even leave New Zealand for a major race. I was really glad I was sick there because they see those symptoms so often they are better able to make an educated guess as to what it is. Whereas I don't think in New Zealand they would have been able to react quickly enough.'

An arduous flight back to Christchurch a few days after he arrived in Singapore completed the worst two weeks of Gurney's life. But there was no instant relief felt at being on home soil. He had lost so much weight and was still so weak that he had to live with his father once he returned. He needed the help and also he couldn't handle the steep gradients that came with his own house. It was utterly soul-destroying for someone so fit, so motivated and so independent to be reduced to this helpless, almost pathetic state. There was worse to follow.

The advice from the medics was that he should knock racing on the head. His body had endured too much stress and the dehydration he would inevitably suffer during these gruelling challenges would not be doing his body any favours. He was still on dialysis once he got back to New Zealand and was required to drink six litres of fluid a day to get his kidneys functioning under their own steam. The trauma for those particular organs had been intense. They had taken enough punishment. It wouldn't be right to put them through real hardship again just for the sake of a race.

The thought of losing his sport made his heart sink. Already emotionally frail, Gurney was almost broken when the letter arrived from his insurance company informing him he owed close to $100,000 for his treatment in Malaysia and Singapore.

'I had some of the worst depression. I thought I would be glad that I survived but coming out of it and reassessing what I would do without my sport … that was so hard. The doctors reckoned I shouldn't have been racing because of the dehydration you suffer on endurance races. I went and talked to some specialists about it and they said sometimes with leptospirosis you get a neurotransmitter imbalance in your nervous system that can cause depression. Also, I had a $92,000 hospital bill to pay off. We ended up getting into a court battle with the insurance company and they paid half of it in the end. But I still had to find $46,000.'

Gurney found himself staring at some pretty stark choices. He could curl into a ball and hope that somehow his life would turn itself around. He could accept the doctors' assessment of his health and agree with them that the risks of racing outweighed the benefits. If he did that, he would one day reach his deathbed and wonder what might have been. Or he could take a more proactive stance. He could be the judge of his own health and take a view that it would be best to wait and see how he recovered. He could make a plan on how he could restore the health of both his body and his bank balance. He could be the master of his own destiny and reach that deathbed knowing he did all he could to reunite with adventure racing.

There was never any question as to which way Gurney would lean. This was a guy who had twice won the world's benchmark multi-sport race. A race that started on Kumara Beach on the West Coast of the South Island and then saw him run a total of 36 km, cycle three stages of 15 km, 55 km and 70 km, and kayak 67 km. A race that would see him arrive on the east coast having travelled a total of 243 km, taking only 11 hours. His two victories had not happened by chance. They had been possible because Gurney was, physically and mentally, one of the toughest humans on the planet. He had been that way since the age of five. His blood had been poisoned in recent weeks but it had not diluted the competitive spirit that coursed through his veins.

'When I first came out of hospital I couldn't even make it to the letterbox,' says Gurney. 'But every day I would set little goals and I would try and walk a few steps further. I was quite surprised at how quickly I recovered. It wasn't that long before I was able to go out on my bike for about an hour or so. I didn't feel strong enough to race fully. That was still a bit of an unknown.

'I didn't want to go too hard. I had been warned not to overdo it after what I had been through. I believed that I could suffer some recurrence from it. I was trying little events. I did the Coast to Coast in 1996 in a celebrity team and I just did the kayak leg.'

A leisurely paddle as part of a team competing for fun didn't offer quite the same thrill as competing against other elite athletes. But it was a start. It was a sign that Gurney was making progress. There was a bit more meat back on his bones. He was that little bit more confident and so much closer to the top end of his sport than he had been 12 months earlier. He was, however, staring at the old cliché of being so near yet so far.

About a year after Gurney's brush with death, Howard was putting a team together for an overseas adventure race. Gurney was keen to be part of it. Howard wasn't. He felt his old pal wasn't ready yet. While he knew Gurney would give everything he had, Howard could see that would not be enough. He could see that Gurney was still short of stamina. He was still short of the conditioning required to take on such demanding races. Howard said no thanks, but he knew next time he would probably not have to reject Gurney again.

'Steve was pretty disappointed but he had lost so much weight and his muscle had all wasted away because of his illness. I didn't think he was ready then, but I always knew he would make it back. Steve never gives up. If we were out on our mountain bikes and we came to a particularly steep section that Steve couldn't cycle up he would go back down and keep trying until he was able to do it. Most other people would just walk with their bikes and then carry on from where they felt they could cycle again. That definitely wasn't Steve's way. He would go back and go back until he could do it.'

And that is effectively what he did for the next year. He went back to training harder and harder. He gradually became more confident that his body would not melt down if he went outside his comfort zone. Every week he got a little stronger. Every week he believed a little more. What he didn't fully appreciate at the time was the new motivation he had. He didn't appreciate how strong a driving force fear had been — the fear that he might never be able to race again. It had fortified his determination, made him even hungrier to win and to enjoy the moment.

By the time February 1997 rolled around, there was an outside chance of him having a particularly special moment to make sure he enjoyed. He was in the right sort of shape to secure his third Coast to Coast title. His body looked a lot more like that of a potential champion. He was thinking exclusively about what he needed to do to win and not worrying about what might go wrong with his body. It was the right formula and he found himself way out in front as he kayaked down the Waimakariri River. He was even further ahead when he got to the finish at Sumner.

'A good look at death really makes you appreciate what you are passionate about. And I think the risk of having my sport taken off me made me even more passionate. I don't recall a dawning moment. I just kept pushing a little bit harder and kept giving more and more. A lot of it was mental. The first six months after I got home were really depressing.

'So I was over the moon when I won the Coast to Coast. It was my best win and proved I was okay again. My self-confidence grew as a result and I think that was my favourite win. It brought tears to my eyes when I took the lead in the kayaking leg and I thought, "Yeah, no one is going to catch me now."'

It was a thought Gurney was going to have every February for the next six years. He won a record seven Coast to Coast titles in a row, taking his total to nine. He was right: no one was going to catch him. Only his age could do that. As Howard says: 'That win in 1997 showed Steve was back. Once I knew he was going to live, I always knew he would get back to racing. It was never my goal to get him back to winning Coast to Coasts. It was my goal to keep him alive. It was an incredible achievement to regain his fitness after being so sick. To get back to winning the Coast to Coast was just amazing. There are probably only about 10 guys, if that, who have done it [i.e. won the Coast to Coast]. The way he saw his life draining away in Malaysia I think gave him the drive to go and win seven Coast to Coasts. I think it made him realise how important racing and his sport were to him.'

His near-death experience did help Gurney realise how much he wanted to race and more importantly, how much he wanted to win. It took him some time, though, to realise that. It also took him some time to fully understand all the things he had to learn from his illness.

He had always known that he was driven. He had known from the time he went to primary school that he felt good about himself when he won things. He knew that he wanted to win things. But he'd never fully understood why it was so important to him. The depression that followed his illness helped him with the answer. The fact he was alive should have been reason to rejoice. Waking up and looking across the Canterbury Plains to see the looming Southern Alps should have been reason enough to keep him smiling. But being alive without being able to compete at his chosen sport left him empty. The power of his emotions made him realise how much he was defined as a person by his sport.

'I have asked the question, "Why do I need to race? Why do I need to win?" I think I am trying to prove something to myself and to the world. I think I am trying to prove that I am good enough. That is why I went back and won seven in a row – I still felt I had to go back and prove something.'

With a grand total of nine Coast to Coast titles to his name, it is hard to imagine how Gurney could have proven himself more emphatically.

Steve Gurney was arguably New Zealand's premier multi-sport, adventure racer. Not only did he win nine Coast to Coast titles between 1990 and 2003, he also won major events in South East Asia, Europe, Australia and Africa. He has been responsible for the invention of some groundbreaking equipment such as the Evolution kayak, which is now the racing norm in New Zealand, and the fully enclosed cycling pod, which has been subsequently banned from elite racing. He graduated from Canterbury University in 1986 with a Mechanical Engineering degree and he runs his own design company in Christchurch.

13

ALLAN ELSOM

All Black 1952–1955

It was the blackest irony that Allan Elsom survived the Second World War only to have his life almost ended on the rugby field.

Not that Elsom has ever spent too much time dwelling on what happened to him. He's one of life's great survivors. He is definitely not the sort to do self-pity or late-night soul-searching.

Elsom, perhaps because he was born in 1925, is most definitely old school. Tragedy and adversity get met with the stiff upper lip. That's what comes of belonging to a generation that never asked for help and certainly didn't expect it.

The removal of choice shaped Elsom's thinking. When the war broke out in 1939 he was only 14. As soon as he was old enough to sign up he did. He was tasked with looking for enemy submarines in the Pacific Ocean. The way he saw it, he had no choice. It was what was expected. Men did their patriotic duty. They served because it was the right thing to do.

His philosophy was partly shaped by his father, who had lost a leg in the First World War. It was a devastating blow for a young man. But his father returned to New Zealand and bought a farm. Never once did he feel as if life owed him something in return for his leg. Never once did he feel bitter. He simply got on with looking after himself and his family.

So when Elsom broke his neck at Lancaster Park in 1947, he felt he had no choice but to firstly survive, then fully recuperate, then get on with his life. In his mind it really was that simple. But to those looking on from the outside, it was anything but simple. It was reasonably terrifying, in fact.

Elsom, a promising 21-year-old, was playing at centre for the Albion Club in Christchurch. He was a noted crash tackler. A player with a deep love of the rough and tumble.

He can't remember much about the incident. And he has tried. He has had nearly 60 years of trying to piece together what happened that day on the famous old ground. His best guess is that after lining up one of the Teachers College forwards, the crafty so-and-so changed direction. Elsom was committed, already airborne with his destination confirmed and non-negotiable. Physics hasn't come up with a way yet to allow the human form to deviate in mid-air.

If only it had, then Elsom wouldn't have crashed head first into the hip of the opposing player. At least he thinks it might have been a hip. It was definitely something that didn't give all that much as Elsom's only memory is searing pain in his neck.

He knows he has deliberately wiped most of the specifics from his memory. It is the in-built protection mechanism of the brain. If we remembered pain in its true state, women would only ever give birth once.

Or perhaps the truth is that his brain was so badly affected by the collision that it wasn't in adequate shape to collate any of the specific information. It probably went off-line in the immediate aftermath that saw Elsom's head wobble around on its mooring, like a flimsy boat being tossed on an angry sea.

'I went in to tackle one of the opposition and somehow my head hit him straight on and I collapsed. They sent for the ambulance chap,' recalls Elsom. 'I had to hold my head because my neck was wobbling and the pain was horrific. So they eventually got a stretcher out to me and loaded me on. Someone was holding my head. Finally we went round to the ambulance room and the ambulance officer got on the phone and I heard him say, "Look you will have to be quick, he hasn't got much time."

'So an ambulance arrived to take me to the public hospital. They got sandbags and laid me on the bed. They had sandbags on each side of my head so it wouldn't move.' Elsom had dislocated his neck. He'd survived a year of war on the Pacific Ocean but only 50 minutes of club football.

A dislocated neck in 1947 was seriously bad news. It's hardly a laughing matter in 2006, but medical science is far more sophisticated now than it was back then. Elsom was at the mercy of the gods. When the St John's ambulance officer urged his colleagues to get a wriggle on, he wasn't being melodramatic. Death was a serious possibility.

Not that you would know that from Elsom. He knew, despite the agony clouding his mind, he was going to survive and be all right. It was back to that choice thing again. He didn't see that he had one. His options were to survive and make a full recovery, or die. It's hardly a choice.

So when he got to hospital, he immediately got on with the business of recovering. He lay on his bed, with his ever-present sandbags wrapped round his head, and kept himself to himself. There was no moaning. He suffered his pain in silence and kept his mind positive. The only thing his doctors could tell him after about a week was that he was not going to die. They couldn't, however, be more specific. There was no guarantee he would walk as he did before. And there was absolutely no guarantee that he would ever play rugby again. No one actually said that, but then again, given the damage done to Elsom's neck, it would have been somewhat stating the obvious. But maybe someone should have said so, as it certainly wasn't obvious to Elsom that he was never going to play again. Thoughts of wearing a black jersey flooded his brain. As did thousands of images, action replays if you like, of the tackle that put him in hospital.

'I have thought about it and thought about it and I don't know how that happened. All I know is I went down and my neck was in pain, flopping around. I had just got out of the navy and you know how blasé you get. I think the game was called off.

'I think I have blocked a lot of it out. But I knew I would come right. When I lay in hospital for four weeks, there was this one chap who was moaning and groaning. And they used to say to him, "Look at that footballer, he doesn't open his mouth. He puts up with pain and you have got a trivial little injury and you are disrupting the whole ward." He shut up after that. I was in pain pretty much the whole time.

'I had one of those sliding mattresses. Nowadays they clamp people's necks. My two sandbags kept my head perfectly still. All I had to do was lie there and dream. I always had faith. All I wanted to do was be an All Black. You have got to have dreams. I am a bit of a dreamer. I kept thinking I was going to be back out there training again. I felt elated when they told me I could go home.'

Of course he did. He was 21 years old and desperate to get on with his life. He would have to take it slowly, though. He had been discharged from hospital, but he was still in some pain. Still nowhere near as mobile as he once was. There were plenty of miles to be clocked on recovery road.

Rugby for the time being went into cold storage. He was obviously in no condition to play and his priority was work. Play could come later – maybe.

He had been working as a cabinet-maker prior to his accident but the idea of going back didn't really appeal. Elsom wanted more. He wanted to be his own boss. So he bought a house and slowly began to do it up. It was hard work for a man who wasn't fully mobile. But he persevered and when he finished and sold it for considerably more than he paid for it, he knew he had found his vocational calling. Elsom wanted to be a property tycoon. The ease with which he waltzed into a new career was an encouraging sign that he could put the events of Lancaster Park behind him. A dislocated neck couldn't derail him professionally.

A few months after leaving hospital and the pain had receded. He was confident in his new work and somewhere in the back of his head a little torch continued to burn for a sport he desperately loved. That light would flicker from time to time. It was usually put out on one of the many occasions when he would find himself cradling his neck in an awkward manner, fearful it could all go wrong again. It was an unwelcome habit and one he didn't know how to break. Until his father sat him down and gave it to him straight.

'It took me a while to get better. It was a few months. My friends would come round and pick me up to go out on a Saturday night and they used to jack me up so my head was steady in the back seat of the car. I was gradually getting back into ordinary life. But whenever I had two or three drinks I would revert back to holding my head at a funny angle and walking in a protective manner. Then one day my father said to me, "You look like an idiot when you walk like that." He told me to pull myself together and to start over again.

'I did feel self-conscious but then again I was just happy to be walking. I didn't have to walk like that. I just thought I did. It was hard but I did it. I had to do it. I had to help myself. No one was going to get out and do it for me. I never had self-pity. My father was a very loveable man. He had lost a leg in the First World War. I had a lovely father and he was right to say what he did. I pulled myself together. I immediately stopped doing that.'

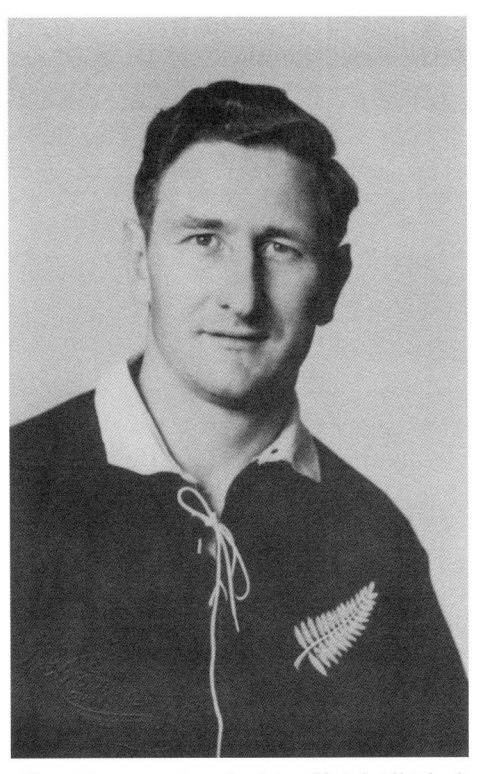

Allan Elsom posing for his official All Black photo in 1952.

As advice goes, this was as to the point as you were ever likely to get. Elsom didn't see it as harsh, though, just honest. It enabled him to move on and leave the accident behind. His business was booming, he was making decent coin. Living with all the trappings a young man should enjoy. Except one – rugby was still not on the agenda. No matter that the torch was still burning, there was uncertainty about a playing return. He'd been out of the game for a few years. His neck, seemingly fully heeled, couldn't be certain to handle the contact. These were different times. There was no state-of-the-art technology to scan his neck and assess the danger. There wasn't a highly experienced physiotherapist on hand to offer an exercise and mobility regime. Elsom was in the dark about the true state of his neck so playing rugby was put in the too hard basket until 1951.

Then his old club came knocking. They asked him to play half a game against the Southern Club from Dunedin. All of a sudden rugby was very much back on the agenda. Most people would have mulled over the invitation. Deliberated with very good reason. When you dislocate your neck playing rugby it takes a very brave man to go back for some more.

Elsom was obviously a very brave man. Once again it was all about choice. If he wanted to avoid the serious irritation of dying wondering, his only option was to get out there and give it a go. Science couldn't give him answers. He could theorise about the chances of his neck being strong enough. He could employ a boffin to work out the odds of something disastrous going wrong. Or he could just take the plunge. In the end he didn't hesitate when the invitation came his way. He said yes as if he had just been asked whether he would like more tea.

Nor did he hesitate when he had to make his first tackle. It was a defining moment for Elsom. A chance to see whether he was the sort of man who confronted his innermost fears or submitted to their debilitating power. He was the former and as it turned out, fortune really did favour the brave.

'I didn't know whether I would play again in those four years. I told myself to keep thinking positively. Subconsciously I probably didn't think I would ever play again. What got me through was that I was confident.

'I played half a game at an Easter tournament and in that game a Canterbury selector walked in and I scored two tries against the Otago centre. The first tackle was very scary. My whole career I was a crash tackler. I used to love it. I was so confident. I used to love pushing the breath out of them. After the first tackle I thought, I'm back into it. I was worried. But when I made that first tackle I was floating. I never thought it would happen again. I had so many injuries through rugby that I never thought about it. I couldn't believe my luck, and it was luck, because the Canterbury selector walked through the gates.'

It wasn't luck that enabled Elsom to score those two tries. That was natural talent. The Canterbury selector could see that, which is why he had no hesitation calling up Elsom for Canterbury's next game. Elsom was 26 but because he had been out of the game for so long no one really knew who he was. That included his Canterbury team-mates. Elsom was aware there was a lot of murmuring and nodding in his direction when he got on the team bus.

It made him self-conscious. It also made him determined to prove he deserved to be there. He didn't want everyone knowing about his neck. That would only make things worse. He was no sympathy selection, getting a reward for being ever so brave. He was there because he was good enough and no matter what his team-mates mumbled to each other about, he was going to win their respect.

'I got picked to play for Canterbury in their annual game against West Coast. I got on the bus and everyone was saying, "Who is that joker? Is he a reporter?" So then I played in that game and scored two tries.

'That was enough for me to get invited on a four-match tour of the North Island. There was this joker Tom Lynch who was the Canterbury centre. He went on the tour to Australia in 1951 with the All Blacks. Our captain Bob Stuart said to Lynch before we played the first game against Manawatu, "This joker Elsom, give him a pass and if he's no good – I have never heard of him – hang on to it." Anyway I scored three tries and before the game ended Bob was shouting out, "For Christ's sake, pass the bloody ball to Elsom." I got a great write-up in the paper. I roomed with Tiny Hill and old Tiny rushed down to get the morning paper and it had a big headline saying a star is born.

'After that I got a knock on the door from a league scout. He wanted me to play league but I refused. But he said, "I tell you what, next year you will be an All Black." I said, "I hope so." '

The scout turned out to be a fairly astute sort of bloke. Elsom did indeed become an All Black in 1952. Following a final trial game in Levin, the New Zealand Press Association reported: 'Elsom, playing on the wing outside Hawke's Bay centre Marett, was the only back to give real thrust to the play. Elsom made ground every time he had the ball and was a constant threat.'

And so it was that Elsom made his test debut against Australia five years after he had dislocated his neck. It was scarcely believable that not so long ago Elsom had lain in the first-aid room at Lancaster Park hearing an ambulance officer speculate he might not have too much longer to live.

On 6 September 1952 he was back at Lancaster Park, wearing black and as sure as ever that he was indestructible. Of course, Elsom never really saw it that way. His neck turned out to be just another injury, albeit a bit more severe and tougher to beat than the many others he encountered. Throughout those four years in the rugby wilderness he never let that torch die. He always believed he could do the impossible and be an All Black.

A victory would have been the perfect ending. But it wasn't to be. The All Blacks lost 14–9 and as a consequence a number of the team, including most of the back line, were dropped for the second test a week later at Athletic Park. Unsurprisingly, as one of life's great survivors, Elsom was selected for another run. Things went a bit better in Wellington and the All Blacks won 15–8.

A year later and he was chosen to tour the UK. For Elsom it was a trip that became memorable for three reasons. The first was that he ended up back in the wars, sustaining the most bizarre injury off the field. Then he was accused of being professional by some crabby English old-boy-network types who got a bit uppity at the fact these damned Colonials were proving to be rather good. The final reason was perhaps more poignant. He was asked to visit a young rugby player who was in hospital after breaking his neck playing rugby. Elsom was living proof that a full and astonishing recovery could be made. So they sent him in to do the whole look at me, son, thing.

'We got to England and we would have training runs and go back to the hotel. We would book up a pint of beer. Some of the English officials reckoned we were professionals because we wouldn't pay for our own beer.

'Then we went to Cardiff where I finished up in hospital. We went to a hotel there and I got a cigarette in the eye. The crowds were around us and one chap had a cigarette. Someone turned me around and it went in my eye. I was lucky because I was put in hospital and there was a splendid doctor who was one of the best in the world at the time. He came in about midnight and sorted me out. I was very lucky. I didn't play again for a month.

'I can remember going to hospital again, though. There was a young fullback who had broken his neck. He was a lovely young chap, but he only lived a fortnight. His injury was much worse than mine.'

It was a reminder of just what Elsom had endured and successfully overcome. But there was one more giant twist in this tale. It came in the 1980s long after Elsom had retired with six All Black tests and 16 games to his credit. He was diagnosed with breast cancer, a disease that is very rare in men. There was a horrid sense of déjà vu. Once again, he was told by a doctor that he didn't have long to live. By now he knew the drill. He simply absorbed the information and resolved to carry on regardless. Positive thinking was the only way. He'd been doing it all his life and had no intention of stopping. He knew there was no other choice.

'My doctors said to me you had better get your affairs in order, you have only got about three months. I came home and told my wife. I never thought about it. I just had the treatment and carried on large as life. My wife says to me that I'm an old bugger and because only the good die young, I'm going to live to 100. I got through the treatment and then I got cancer on the other breast. This was very rare for a male. I used to get calls from doctors asking if they could take my file away and talk about it. Some doctors had never seen a male with breast cancer. I have had some ups and downs.'

That's Allan Elsom for you. Master of the chronic understatement and a man who typifies all that is good about a generation that grew up adamant they were owed nothing.

Allan Elsom played six tests and 16 games for the All Blacks, scoring three points from a dropped goal in the 8–0 win against Australia at Carisbrook in 1955. Elsom became a key figure in the Canterbury side that held the Ranfurly Shield between 1953 and 1956, with his rugged defence considered one of the red and blacks' most fearsome weapons. He also shored up the Canterbury midfield that claimed back-to-back victories against the Springboks and All Blacks in 1956 and 1957. He retired from first-class rugby in 1958 at the age of 33. He went on to enjoy a successful career in property development and splits his time between Christchurch and Akaroa. He is 80.

14

JEFFREY THUMATH

New Zealand Athletics Junior Representative and Sprint Champion

Normally, being seen naked by your mum would not be considered a good thing. In some cases it could even constitute the sort of disaster from which you never fully recover.

For 17-year-old Jeffrey Thumath it was the best thing that ever happened to him. His mother walked in on him changing one day and caught sight of his fiercely distended testicle. She had him whisked to Accident & Emergency before he'd even had time to stop blushing. Thumath didn't bother to protest. Doing the whole outrage thing wasn't going to cut any ice and besides, a few hours after arriving at hospital he was told he had testicular cancer.

If his mum had not walked in when she did, Thumath would probably never have been standing on the long jump runway at Ericsson Stadium 12 months later about to break a 38-year-old junior record. If his mother's intrusion had happened in April 2002, rather than March 2002, the tumour in Thumath's body would almost certainly have found its way to his brain. As it was it had made its way from his testicle, to his stomach and up to his chest. He was diagnosed as having Stage 3 testicular cancer. That was not great news.

Testicular cancer is very treatable – if caught early. For those who present in Stage 1 – where the tumour is confined to the testicle – the chances of recovery are 98 per cent. They drop significantly at Stage 2 when the cancer has spread to the stomach. By the time they get into the lungs – Stage 3 – 50-50 is about as optimistic as the doctors ever get. Those unfortunate enough to develop to Stage 4 are left clinging to a cliff face that affords little purchase.

The prognosis for Thumath was nearly as bad as it could have been. His saving grace was that the cancer had not spread to his brain. Being young and fit were also plus factors.

But probably the most important factor that led him back to the track was his unflappable demeanour. His thoughts never strayed from the positive. And there were plenty of ill winds trying to buffet him into a destiny he was far too young to fulfil. He had been struck down in the prime of his life. That was reason enough to be bitter. Then there was the fact he had always looked after himself. In January 2002 he had been to the New Zealand National Athletic Championships and won the Junior long jump title. He'd also recorded respectable times in both the 100 m and 200 m to get among the medals. To win at that level, he'd lived his life very much on the straight and narrow. The temptations that were too much for other teenagers didn't get their claws into Thumath. To play by the rules and be dealt such a harsh blow was hardly fair.

It seemed he was being punished for living in the West Auckland suburb of Massey. It was possibly coincidence, possibly not, that other Massey teenagers were also being struck down with cancer at the same time. It was possibly coincidence, possibly not, that two of them lived on the same street as Thumath. And it was possibly coincidence, possibly not, that a disproportionately high volume of power pylons run through Massey.

One of those other teenagers was Cameron Duncan, who became nationally famous for making a powerful short film. Duncan, a close friend of Thumath's, lost his battle with cancer. The other was Charles Hetaraka, a softball player who was generally thought to be on his way towards making the national team. Just like Duncan, Hetaraka met his maker at an appallingly young age. Thumath didn't need to look for reasons to be angry. They were in his face.

But that wasn't his approach. Prior to his diagnosis his dream was to represent New Zealand at the Commonwealth and Olympic Games. He was, arguably, the most promising long-jumper in the country. He was also a more than capable sprinter, particularly over 200 m. His goals were realistic and getting cancer wasn't going to change any of that.

'I was in a period in my life where I was just relaxing in my seventh form. Then I was diagnosed with testicular cancer. I had an operation the next day. With the tumour being the size it was I didn't have a clue what it could be. I didn't even know the symptoms. Mum came in one day when I was changing and said, "We are going to Accident & Emergency." That was it. That was my normal life over. I had surgery. The doctor pretty much knew straight away. I had about a week off to recover and then I was into chemotherapy. There were tumours in my stomach and lungs. They were hoping it wasn't in my brain, which it wasn't. So that was a major relief. It was pretty scary stuff.

'My immediate thoughts were that I wanted to get back into my sport and back into my life. I had been pretty successful at athletics. I had been named in the New Zealand Junior team. Everything was looking promising and then I was struck down with cancer. But I said, "I'm not going to let this stop me." I said, "I'm going to get back to where I was and achieve everything I wanted." '

One of the first things he wanted to achieve when – and with Thumath it was always when, never if – he put his cancer behind him, was to win the senior boys' long jump at the 2003 Auckland Secondary Schools Championships. The competition was a year away. For Thumath it would be the toughest year he had ever endured. Which is why, come March 2003, when his foot landed perfectly on the board, he was propelled by a most potent cocktail of emotions. Everything he had endured in the last 12 months was condensed into one explosive leap.

Relief formed a significant part of the cocktail – relief that he had been right all along to believe he could return to his normal life. His faith was shaken by the severity of the physical toll the disease and treatment extracted. He was in superb shape around the time of his diagnosis. His lean frame was weighted perfectly with a trim finish of muscle. He was ever so nicely balanced at 75 kg.

But a few months later and he looked like he had just staggered out of Belsen, the infamous Nazi concentration camp. That was hardly surprising. For a start he had endured reasonably traumatic surgery. That was unpleasant, but not a patch on the chemotherapy – which is medicine's equivalent of napalm. Doctors effectively drop the chemo drugs into a vein and then run for cover. They know these drugs don't take any prisoners. Thumath's weight plummeted to 62 kg. His strength evaporated like spilled petrol on a sunny day and he began to wonder if he would ever make it back to the track. By the end of his fourth and final chemotherapy cycle he was gasping on the ropes. His body really didn't look like it would even be able to propel itself from the board into the pit.

The last thing he needed to learn at that point was that he had a mature teratoma tumour growing inside his stomach. The teratoma was benign but continuing to grow by leeching Thumath's blood. By the time it was discovered, the tumour measured 16 cm by 19 cm. It had to be removed, which required some more brutal surgery.

He was excruciatingly frail by the end of 2002 when he resumed training for real. It would be a long way back. A very long way back. He was competing in explosive sports. His legs needed to generate dramatic power to first carry him down the runway at electrifying speed and then propel him up and forward. It takes sprinters and jumpers years of work in the gym and track to generate the elasticity and strength required in their core muscle groups. Thumath could in time regain the bulk and muscle fibre that he had lost, but it would be an agonising slog. He would be way behind his peer group.

At that stage, though, his athletics career was more of a secondary concern. The advanced nature of his cancer had put his life in real and present danger. He may have been focused on getting back into his sport but his family could see that survival had to be the primary objective. His body had been ravaged. That was disappointing and produced a multitude of frustrations. But if he had fallen into a mire of self-pity at his vastly reduced athletic capacity, he would have been failing to see the much bigger picture. So no matter how much hard work loomed for Thumath in his quest to regain his former physique and recapture his speed and agility of old, the most important thing for him to grasp was that the medics were pleased with his progress. They were comfortable that he was beating the disease. He may have looked like a one-iron with ears, but the worst was behind him. The weekly grind of having poison pumped inside him was gone, so too the constant nausea. The tiredness was subsiding and he was gradually building his strength to the point where simply sitting up didn't seem such a chore any more. He needed to be thankful for these not so small mercies.

Not only had his body been decimated by two bouts of surgery and four rounds of chemotherapy, he had also been unable to train seriously for almost nine months. It certainly didn't make his life any easier that, when he returned, he had to train on his own for much of the time as his immune system couldn't handle any infection.

Training with others was a risk, so the hard slog had to be done solo. There would be no one for him to chase and no one to spur him on in those agonising last sprints of every session. There would be no one to push him through the pain barrier. A barrier that was a lot lower than it had been a year ago.

'It was really hard to get the conditioning back. I couldn't be near anyone who was sick because my immune system was screwed. When I first came back I was only able to do a fraction of the training because my body was so weak. It took months to get back into it.

'I had heard the stories about chemo and how terrible it was. But I wasn't worried about the side effects. I knew my hair would come back. It was the sickness that I didn't really want. The vomiting and being weak, I didn't really like being weak. Being struck down and confined to bed was pretty tough. I'm a very active person.

'Each week I was going in to have my chemo, I was having blood tests that day to see if I was okay to have chemo. Each week I was borderline. I was just okay to have my chemo. They gave me a VO2 test for my

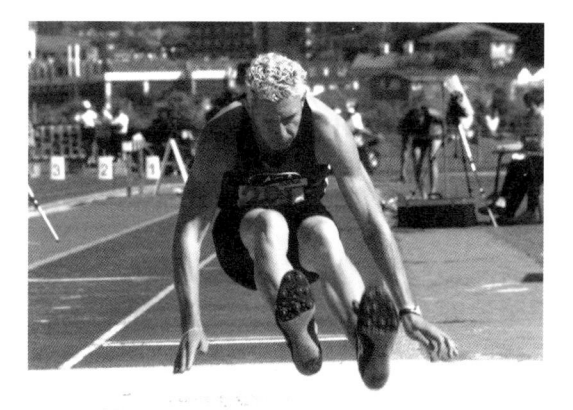

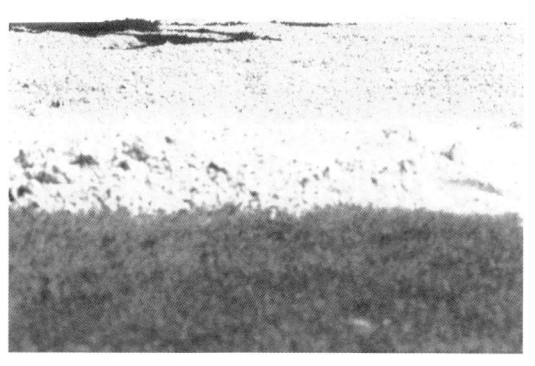

Jeffrey Thumath in action at the National Championships in Dunedin, 2003.

lungs before the chemo and after. They couldn't understand that my results were as good after as they were before even though I had the Bleomicin, a drug in the chemotherapy that scars your lungs.

'I suppose I also looked at it as a really good rest. It was months of resting my body. I had been doing a lot of work since I was 15 and my body came back a lot quicker and developed in a way that was stronger. Since then I have been in the best shape of my life.'

He wasn't just physically stronger, either. By the time he leapt into the humid Auckland air in March 2003, he was mentally tougher than any teenager should have been. Staring at death had formed a steely core. Seeing good friends die had hardened him to the harsh reality that life is not fair. Fate will not necessarily smile on the good. Thumath learned, that just for the sheer hell of it, fate could be a bitch. Cancer helped him understand that he was owed nothing. It helped him understand how much he wanted to succeed and also that the onus to succeed lay with him and him alone.

His disease had taken him to the brink. As the chemo bubbled in his blood he would have occasional doubts about his ability to make it back. There would be fleeting moments when he was physically drained that he would wonder whether he would ever be able to achieve the goals he was setting himself every day. The idea of even making it to the take-off board seemed ambitious enough at times.

'I had no idea at that point whether I was going to come back or not. I knew I had a positive attitude and that I wanted to get back into it, but I didn't know how long it would take. I had goals each day and I had goals for my athletics. I didn't know how long it would take to recover. I didn't know if I could recover my strength. It was just the not knowing that was so hard.

'Everything happened so fast it didn't really hit me until a month or two later when I was having my chemo and I couldn't see my friends. That's when it really shocked me because it was not a normal life for a 17-year-old.

'There was one time in hospital when I said, why me? I had a little chemo reaction and I had to be in hospital for a week. It was just one night where I had to be alone and my brother had called from England. I did say, what's the point? But the next day I was over it. It was a little thing, maybe a five-second thing of not believing.'

Those doubts were only fleeting. They were always submerged shortly after surfacing. Sunk by more buoyant positive thoughts. His coach, Paul Lothian, could scarcely believe his protégé was seriously ill, so powerful was Thumath's sunny demeanour.

'Jeff's chemo didn't seem to worry him in the slightest. He had one day where he was crook, the rest of the time he was fine. I used to go up and see him in the hospital and he would be lying there and we would talk. You wouldn't have thought there was much wrong with him at all. He actually used to come and do a little bit of training when he was going through his chemo.

'It never crossed my mind that he wouldn't come back. I just assumed he would toss it off and return to his sport. Jeff was able to put all the cancer stuff to one side. He said he just wanted to train and that he didn't want to talk about all that other stuff. He has been able to overcome massive problems.'

What Thumath took from his cancer experience was the belief that he had steered himself through the most treacherous path and that he was now equipped with the emotional skills to achieve all his life goals.

Before his diagnosis he had been drifting through his final year at

Massey High School without any grand plan as to what he would do next. The realisation that he had maybe been given a second chance at life focused his mind both on the track and off it. He enrolled at Auckland University of Technology to study for a diploma in sport and recreation. Cancer had made him a better person, more rounded and determined to succeed. And with that came an inner peace. An inner peace brought about by the knowledge he was actively taking charge of his own destiny. The trick to that was setting goals as he charged over the top of his illness.

He couldn't afford to be aimless during his treatment. His mind needed targets. Every day in hospital he would set himself a goal. It gave him a hunger he had never experienced before. He became desperate to break that Auckland Secondary Schools' long jump record. What better way to announce his triumph over his disease? The hunger began to burn as much as the poisons.

That hunger became so fierce it even forced him to compete at the national championships at the end of 2002 just weeks after his surgery and last bout of chemotherapy. He wasn't even in the right ball-park in terms of conditioning, but after weeks in hospital, and weeks of vomiting and tiredness, Thumath knew exactly how much athletics meant to him. He didn't do weak and helpless very well. All those weeks of just lying there feeling drained and hopeless in his hospital bed had hammered home how much he loved being out on the track. When athletics was taken off the agenda, he learned fully how much he wanted it put back on. Those months of inactivity and sickness had fortified his ambition and his competitive streak emerged from his ordeal more oak tree than sapling.

'It would have been very hard not to have come back. Even if I were injured, I would want to run. That year I was diagnosed, I went to the Nationals and I wasn't meant to compete. I went as a manager for the school. We got down there and I walked on the track and thought, no, I have to run here. I phoned Mum and got her to send down my spikes and all my gear. They got me into the meeting a night before the race. All my mates asked me what I was doing there. I wasn't meant to compete but I had to. It was the instinct, the will to win, the passion for racing that forced me out there. I came out of chemo in June and had my operation in September. I had three months off

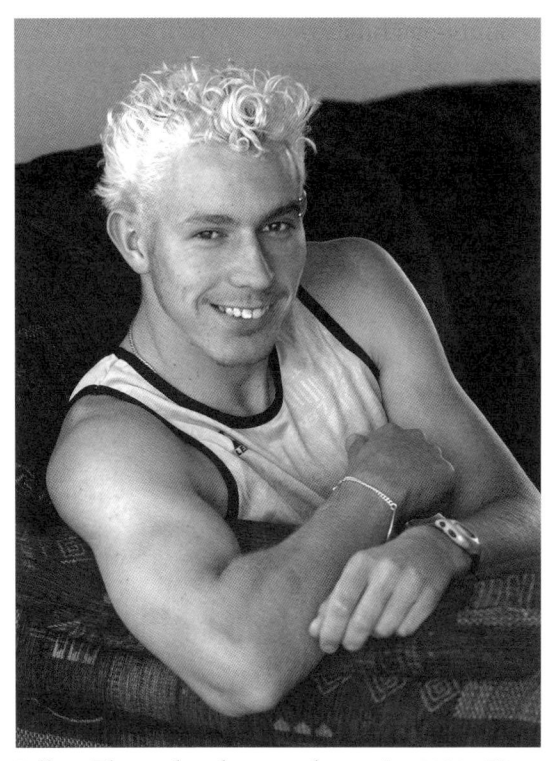

Jeffrey Thumath relaxes at home in 2004. *Fiona Goodall, Suburban Newspapers*

and went to the Nationals that year. I hadn't recovered and I hadn't trained but I wanted to get the afterburners out. I came fifth equal in the long jump and made semifinals in the 100 m. I was pretty stoked about that.

'My athletics goals were very important. I wanted to go to the Olympics and the Commonwealth Games. I didn't know what year. I was looking at the 2006 Commonwealth Games in Melbourne. Now I have set my goals back.

'I didn't know what I was going to do once I left school. I didn't know if I was going to go to university or not. In a way I was just relying on my sport and I reckon the cancer helped me to become more determined. I turned out to be a better person for it. I wasn't really thinking about my future as such. I was just going to school and eating my lunch. Not really studying. Because of what happened I have had time to sit down and think what I want to do with my life outside athletics.'

The other big factor that drove him was the need for closure. He'd spent a year of his life fighting cancer and as a consequence it had redefined him. But he needed to embark on a new chapter to make the struggle of the previous year worth while. There needed to be a landmark to formally announce the closure of his cancer life and the re-opening of his normal life.

Smashing the record at the Auckland Secondary Schools by 17

centimetres was just the start. From there he could attack his next goal and keep proving he was a better, stronger athlete than he was pre-cancer.

'In February 2003 I went to the Auckland Secondary School qualifiers and got close to the record in the senior boys' long jump. A week later in the finals I ended up breaking that 38-year-old record. The record was 7.09 m and I jumped 7.26 m. That was also a personal best. Once I broke it I wanted to go to the nationals and get either a record or a medal. I went to Dunedin and competed in the Under-18, Under-20 and senior long jump. I won two bronze medals and a gold. I was stoked. I felt like I was getting back on track. In April I applied for a trip to Darwin. I got it. I came back with four gold medals and a silver medal in an international meet.

'What was important was I felt like that jump at the Auckland Secondary Schools gave me closure. Then I went to the Australian Under-23 championships in Sydney and qualified for the World Juniors in the 200 m with 21.29 seconds. I didn't think I would ever make it and I did. I had been thinking about the 100 m and long jump but I qualified in the 200 m. It was a bit weird for the World Juniors as four of us qualified. Because only three of us could run in the 200 m we had to have a race off. I was slightly injured so I didn't run. I still went to the championships in Italy and ran in the 4x100 m relay and we came twelfth. We just missed out on making the final by 0.2 seconds so we were a bit peeved.'

The lonely hours training with only his own shadow for company had reaped a reward richer than he had ever imagined. Barely strong enough to make it from his bed to the toilet at the peak of his chemo, here he was now running times that put him in the company of the best young sprinters in the world. That stick-thin, withered shell that he had been only months back seemed to be a ghost that no one could quite recall.

Certainly no one could equate the Thumath they saw in June 2002 with the one they saw gliding round the track in June 2003. The former carried the torpid stench of illness and looked for all the world as if he might dissolve in a heavy rain shower. The other looked to be the emerging face of New Zealand athletics. He had that air of success all champions faintly emanate without ever realising. His times were impressive. So too his haul of medals that had been won in gifted company. He was, literally, back on track. His belief and perseverance could yet be rewarded with a trip to an Olympic Games. That remains the ultimate dream. The odds are shorter on him making it to the Commonwealth Games, assuming he is able to recover from what will hopefully be the final stage in his cancer ordeal.

Just as he was building some impressive momentum, there was yet more bad news to be delivered. Presumably Thumath unwittingly signed up for his bad luck module to be taken all at once. If not, and if his luck continues to be quite aggressively unfortunate, he might have to start wondering whether he committed some heinous crimes in a former life.

His progress was halted during the 2005-2006 season when it was discovered that he had two more mature teratomas. The original surgery in his stomach had only removed 90 per cent of the tumour, with his medical team hoping the remainder would simply die away naturally. It didn't happen and the tumour grew to 10 cm by 11 cm, with another measuring 10 cm by 9 cm on his right lung. Both had a five-year window where they could turn cancerous. The surgery, which took place at the end of 2005, was serious. Significantly, the debilitating nature of the tumours was also reasonably serious and yet Thumath was still competing and continually breaking his personal bests. Once Thumath rehabilitates, it will be the first time in almost four years that he has been able to run with a clean bill of health. And Lothian can't hide his excitement at the prospect of seeing Thumath return to training with no medical hindrance. The last few years have only made his athlete stronger.

'There is no reason he can't make the Commonwealth Games and I'm pretty hopeful that he still can. He was jumping 7.26 m before his last round of surgery and if he can get up to 7.80 m or 7.90 m that should get him to the Commonwealth Games. I think that is realistic for him. In the 200 m if he can run 20.5 seconds that would get him away. If he sets his mind to something he will achieve it. He has that ability.'

And if Thumath does indeed make it to New Delhi in 2010 he will not need any reminding of how special that will be. He's reviewed the events of 2002 again and again and is fully aware of the fine line he straddled. On one side was a rich and rewarding life. A life where he could wear a black vest with a silver fern and feel his heart almost bursting with pride. On the other was a horrid, tragic death, probably before his 19th birthday. He saw good friends Cameron Duncan and Charles Hetaraka fall on the wrong side.

He knows he was lucky. He played his part by fighting every inch, but with cancer, particularly Stage 3 testicular cancer patients who survive, there is always an element of luck. That's not something he will ever forget.

'I feel I have been given a second chance. But in a way it is all to do with determination and all the support I have had from my friends and family. All your mates want to see you get back. That gives you the incentive to get back into normal life. To get back to how you were before your diagnosis.

'My cancer will always be with me. It is there. I just don't dwell on it. What is in the past is in the past. It may affect me in later life. I'm looking at what I can achieve with what I have got. I am here, but if I hadn't been caught changing by Mum when I was – if I had left it another two weeks – I wouldn't be here. That was how close I was to dying. I have moments when I think, thank God. I didn't actually realise how close I was until Mum told me that the doctor actually said that about the two weeks. I thought back and thought I was really lucky that Mum walked in when she did.' There really can't be many teenagers who feel the same way about being caught in the buff by their mother.

Jeffrey Thumath got the go-ahead to resume full training in January 2006 after he had two mature teratomas removed. He hopes to make it to the 2008 Olympics and 2010 Commonwealth Games as either a sprinter or a long-jumper or even both. He has run 10.66 seconds for the 100 m, 21.29 seconds for the 200 m and jumped 7.36 m for the long jump. He has represented New Zealand at the World Junior Games and has won the 100 m in both the junior and senior divisions at the New Zealand Secondary Schools Championships. He has won the Under-18 and Under-20 long jump titles at the New Zealand Championships and has also won medals in these divisions in both the 100 m and 200 m. He recently completed his diploma in sport and recreation and has enrolled for a diploma in fitness training. He lives in Auckland.

15

JARED LOVE

Robert Holden Memorial Winner, Paeroa, 2005

When the paramedic came flying out the back of the ambulance, it was the most disturbing paradox. The ambulance officer had been expelled by the seriously injured Jared Love. But that didn't make any sense at all. The odds on the seriously injured Love surviving to the end of the day were only 15 per cent. Could he really be capable of physical assault? Well, yes, he could. Love, after all, was fighting for his life. Literally.

Love had suffered a massive brain trauma and had not the first clue what he was doing. His frantic lashing was, as odd as it may seem, a natural reaction. Serious brain traumas tend to push their victims down one of two paths. The first is into a docile, almost comatose state. The other sees the victim lash out in the most aggressive manner. Love had gone down the second path. He was thrashing away in the back of the ambulance, kicking and punching those people who were desperately trying to save his life. It didn't exactly make things easy. If Love had known he was making his own skin hard to save, he would have stopped in an instant. But then again maybe he wouldn't have. He had plenty to be angry about.

It was February 2000 and the 23-year-old Love was a week away from flying to Europe to fulfil his sporting dream. He had signed a contract to ride with Yamaha Switzerland. He was on the edge of the big time. If he could cut the mustard in Switzerland, his ticket to the World Superbike Series would surely come. Love had all the talent. He had the necessary fortitude to sit on a motorbike travelling at speeds in excess of 200 km per hour. And he had that ultra streamline focus required to steer a young man away from potential distractions. It was just a matter of time before he showed the world he was brave enough and good enough to compete with the best.

But he had one more thing to do before heading off to Switzerland. He had to ride at Paeroa in the famous street race. It was for old times' sake. New Zealand had given him his start in the sport. There had been some generous sponsors who had gone above and beyond the call of duty. Paeroa was an opportunity to sign off on a high. There was no better way to reward all the financial backers who had supported him than by giving them a victory in his final outing in New Zealand.

But Love wasn't so sure. He was coming under pressure from his team in Switzerland not to ride. Street racing doesn't have the greatest reputation when it comes to safety. Love was reluctant to go, but his father, Laurie, felt his son would be doing the right thing by racing. Jared's sponsors and fans would expect to have one last chance to see him in action. Paeroa was an iconic race and it needed the support of the big-name riders. Once Love senior made the suggestion, the noises of discontent lessened.

Laurie Love, himself a talented rider, was his son's hero. He was both Jared's manager and his mentor. Going to Paeroa was the right call. But by 9 am on the morning of the race, Laurie Love would have given anything for the chance to go back in time and persuade his son to stay in Hamilton that day.

'In the week before the race Jared had a lot of pressure coming from Europe not to race. But once I persuaded him he came round. He said he would do it, but he didn't want to go over there to be embarrassed. He said he was going there to win. But the day before he took his bike out for a warm-up and it dropped a valve just as he was driving it in the street. That made him change his mind again, but I said we had a spare engine and we could sort it out. He went to bed saying he wasn't going to go but he soon cooled down.

'When we got to Paeroa, though, and we were setting up in the pits, we couldn't find the power for a long time. I got the power on quite late to get the tyre warmers going. From our information, the production bikes were going to be the first out. But that all changed and they decided that superbikes would be up first. We had only had the tyre warmer on for about five or 10 minutes which is nowhere near enough. You need about half an hour. And the road temperature was very cold as it was early in the morning. So when Jared went out I said, "For God's sake take it easy."

'He did. I saw him go by a couple of times weaving all over the road to try and warm up the tyres. I saw him and I thought, that's cool. Then one of the top riders came into the pit lane on his bike and he yelled at me that Jared was hurt bad and that I had better get up there.'

Hurt bad didn't come close. Love was critical. To this day no one is sure exactly what caused him to come off his bike backwards. Not even the man himself.

'It wasn't raining. I was doing maybe 50 km. They reckon the track temp was cold. It could have been the cold slicks, it could have been a number of things. I must have spun round and been flipped off. Maybe I landed on the kerb. No one can really tell. You just hear a million different stories.

'What I can remember is I was really frustrated at how the season had gone. I had had a realistic chance of winning the championship but I had blown five motors. I said to Dad I didn't want to go to Paeroa. My family is not rich and Dad had mortgaged the house and loaned me the $60,000 I needed to secure my ride in Switzerland. We had jacked the ride up and sussed everything out. It was a good ride. I was 23 and had been given all this money for a shot. I was shitting myself. I was scared and excited. It was the European rounds of the world superbike series. I would have been riding in a professional environment and learning an enormous amount.

'But Dad said to go to Paeroa and have one last ride before I went to Europe. It was a great chance to have one last scrap with Tony Rees, a legend of racing. I remember doing one and a half laps and then, I don't know. I landed on the back of my head. I split my helmet open, dislocated my skull, separated my brain, cracked my C1 and C2 vertebrae

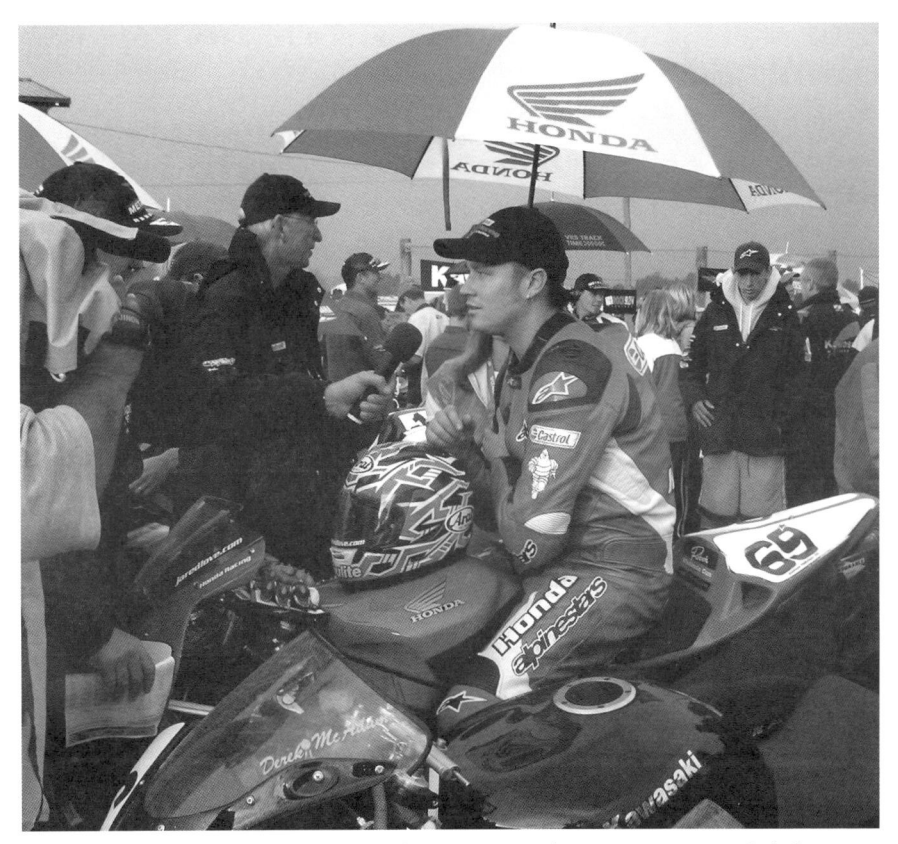

Jared Love is interviewed prior to the VK300 Endurance race at Pukekohe, May 2005. *Terry Stevenson*

and popped my lungs. I was in a bad way. Everyone stood back bar one person – Jason McEwen. He came up beside me and shouted for someone to hold his bike. He whipped my helmet off and checked my airways. Unfortunately Dad had to watch it.'

Laurie Love arrived at the ambulance just as the paramedic came flying out the back. His son was convulsing and it was then that Love senior knew just how grave the situation was. The day had veered off-plan from the instant the sun came up. Now, though, it had taken an appalling detour. Whoever was writing the script had maybe overdone the element of catastrophe. This was a young man with everything to live for being asked to show how hard he was prepared to fight for everything he had.

Or maybe it wasn't a test of resolve. Maybe Love was simply being dealt the crappy hand he had so far managed to avoid.

Love came to Paeroa without having tasted failure. His natural talent for sport had seen him succeed at whatever he turned his hand to. His first medals came in badminton, a sport encouraged by his mother on account of its reassuringly low injury rate. Rugby came on to the agenda in his teens and his chronic lack of appreciation for his own personal well-being enabled him to make the top teams.

But really, badminton, rugby and athletics were just about killing time before he was allowed to jump on a motorbike. Bikes were his true love. They were in his blood and at 16, Love took out the New Zealand motocross championships. That was the sport for him until his final year at school when he suffered his third concussion and was forced to stand down from all sport for 12 months. It was a frustrating period for Love, but far from destroying his spirit, it simply confirmed to him that he absolutely had to have motorbikes in his life. The prospect of living without the smell of petrol or the roar of the engine was not one he could contemplate. But a random invitation to try out a road bike at the end of his year in isolation sent him in a slightly different direction.

'I received an invitation to have a trial on a road bike. I got straight on and almost beat the national champion. Racing was in my blood. I loved motocross but then road racing came into my life. I told my dad how fast I was and he pretty much said, whatever. If someone tells me I can't do something it makes me very determined. I really wanted to prove something to Dad.

'So after I had a play on this road bike I went out and bought a $2,500 machine and won the nationals in my first year. I got the top ride for Suzuki and should have won the superbikes in my first year. But I still managed to get a ride with Yamaha Switzerland lined up. Things had gone unbelievably fast. It was a huge learning curve.'

But as Love battled for his life at Paeroa, the chances of him going to Switzerland weren't looking great. He'd been riding an incredible wave all the way into Paeroa and now it had crashed, spilling him on to the street with a sickening force. He'd come off his bike before. Never, though, with such severity. When Love senior got to his son, the scenario didn't make great viewing.

'I ran to where the ambulance was. I got to the back of the ambulance and he was convulsing. The ambulance guys were trying to administer drugs to calm him down and the chopper was on its way. That was really hard to take. One of the ambulance guys came out on his backside and landed on the bumper. Jared had kicked the poor guy out and he picked himself up and went back in there like he was ready to face a bull. They were really trying to calm him down. As far as Jared was concerned, he was in a fight for his life.

'Eventually they managed to subdue him enough to get him into the helicopter. All the paramedics were looking at their watches because they wanted to get him to Hamilton within the magic hour. Jared and his girlfriend were loaded in and they flew off. They said it was imperative that he didn't have another fit of rage in the helicopter. He started to be sick and that was another sign they didn't like. With about five minutes to go to the hospital one of the paramedics asked the pilot how long it would be before they landed. The pilot said, "About five minutes," and the paramedic replied, "The sooner the better I think mate. It's not good."

'If there was the remotest possible chance he would pull through I knew he would. I had a confident feeling, but by the same token it was out of my hands.'

The panic was rising, but Laurie Love had to stay calm. He had to gather up the gear and trust the medics. As he scrambled round the pit lane, he had to endure ill-informed rumour about the death of his son. It was a severe test of his faith. He knew his boy was still alive. He knew Jared was fighting, but there was no communication with the helicopter as it flew from Paeroa to Hamilton. Could it be that Jared had died on the way? Could it be the rumour was in fact the latest truth?

It was a horrid time. Love had been classified a Status Two, which effectively means he was rated about a 15 per cent chance to survive. Those odds weren't great. They certainly weren't good enough to stop Laurie thinking the worst as he sped back to Hamilton. As he drove he was

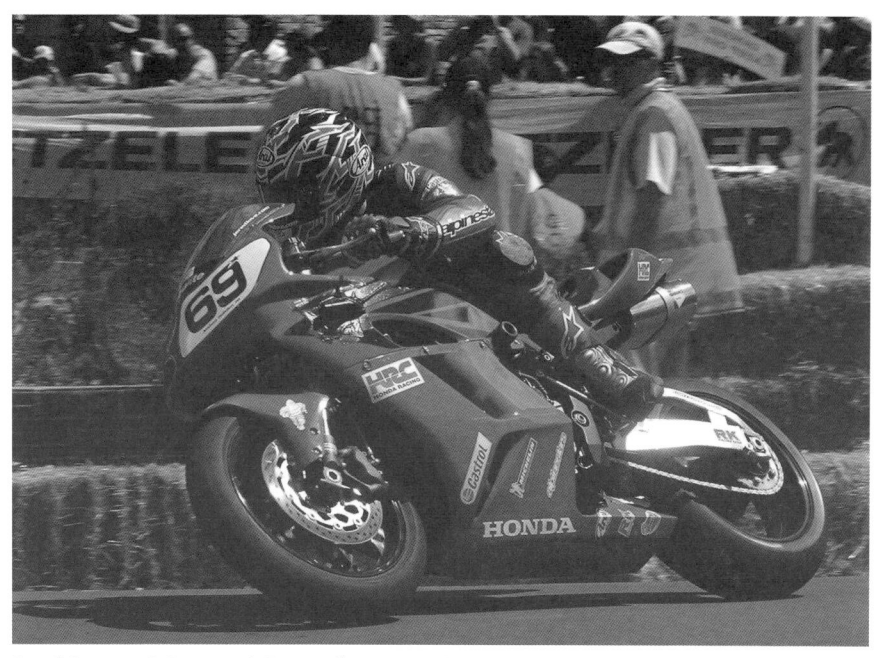

Jared Love at Wanganui, December 2005. *Terry Stevenson*

clinging to that hope buried deep inside him that if there was a chance, his son would stay alive.

'I knew he was okay when he flew away. I got over to Waikato Hospital as quickly as I could. I got a phone call from my other son who had got to the hospital. He was very emotional and said that Jared had landed and he wasn't good. When I got there I couldn't see him. It was a matter of waiting. They had him on a life support system in the Intensive Care Unit. At about 8.30 pm that night we were allowed in to see Jared.

'The doctor told us Jared was sedated. He was acting extremely violently as soon as they turned the support off. The doctor said there are two things. He said, "Jared is either really gone and he's a vegetable or he's fighting for his life." He said at that stage they couldn't tell. He asked me to help by holding Jared's hand and hold him down. This registrar then shouted at Jared. He said, "Jared can you hear me?" Jared squeezed my hand and the registrar had a big grin and said he was going to be fine. About 20 minutes later Jared became conscious and he said, "How's my bike?"'

Death would not be visiting Jared Love. He'd survived, yet there was still no way of knowing how severe a toll the crash had taken. The initial examinations were encouraging. Physically he was bruised and sore – a fairly miraculous return. Mentally, though, there would be no real way of telling what sort of shape he was in until a bit further down the track. His brain had taken the sort of wallop it should never take. There would be short-term implications such as memory loss, anxiety and loss of appetite. If things were really bad, there was the prospect of long-term depression and reduced mental capacity.

Sadly, none of this was fully explained to Love, as once he came out of the ICU onto the general ward, his standard of care plummeted. He effectively slipped through the net and was allowed to return home after a couple of days with no real understanding of what his life would be like.

'When they tried to wake me up, I woke up no sweat. I concussed myself that hard that I pretty much lobotomised myself. I had short-term memory loss and loss of appetite. But they got me there within the magic hour and there was no bleeding. I can remember writing a note when I woke up. It read: "This mouthpiece sucks. When did I crash? Is the bike fucked?"

'After a couple of days the doctors said, "Do you want to go home?" Once I got home the TV show *Rescue One* came out and interviewed me. They showed me footage of the crash and I thought, "Holy shit, why didn't anyone tell me about the crash?" I kept forgetting. I didn't know I had a head injury. I was punch drunk. I was munted.'

But little did Love realise that surviving the crash had been the easy bit. His life was not going to neatly drop back into place. There was his contract with the Swiss team for a start. That had to be canned. He had been due in Europe the week after Paeroa. Clearly that wasn't going to happen. No one could say when he would be able to race again. It was maybe even a case of if rather than when. He needed to pass psychometric tests to regain his licence. And that wasn't proving easy.

Not being able to race ripped at his soul. Bikes were his life. The relationship between Love and his bike, the appropriately numbered 69, aka the Love Machine, had transcended beyond man and machine. Having sat atop the Love Machine for so long, almost by a process of osmosis, the throbbing power of the bike's engine had infiltrated Love. Man and machine were as one. The enforced separation was excruciating.

That wasn't the worst of it, either. Love wasn't allowed to work for a year. His pre-crash existence was comfortable. There was good money coming in. Post-accident he had to survive on a benefit. And still that wasn't the worst of it. Just when he needed the warm bosom of his loved ones the most, his support network collapsed. His girlfriend of four years left him. She may as well have ripped his heart out and tossed it in the bin on her way out the door. Then his father, the man he trusted and respected the most, revealed he was having an extra-marital affair.

'They were my two best friends. The three of us travelled round together. I didn't know if it was the head injury or me going insane but I couldn't tell anybody about what was going on. I didn't want to wreck my dad's life or my mum's. But I had nowhere to turn. That was what was really hurting me.

'My whole life had gone. I had the best parents. They had given me opportunities. They were nice and kind, but I hadn't seen the other side of life. My whole life was whipped out in one day. My girlfriend left me and then Mum found out about Dad. I had a clinical psychiatrist hanging around with me because they say with such a big head injury there is a really high chance of depression. They were worried I was going to kill myself. I had to live on a friend's couch for about four months on $160 a week. I had gone from international superbike ride to no job for a year living in a dude's lounge. Then one of my best mates died of leukaemia on my birthday.

'Losing my girlfriend ripped me. I was telling everyone my accident was nothing. I almost wished that I had died. What was the point keeping me alive for this shit? I was fine with my accident. I counselled everybody. I felt if I had left, I had enjoyed a beautiful life. When I saw my mate die that hurt me very hard. I realised what I had put everyone through.

'It was like here is the cool part of your life and then here is the shit module but all at once. It was too much. I had nobody to talk to in this whole world. I was going to kill myself. I would have just preferred to slip away.'

Getting back on his bike, literally, seemed the only way to bring Love out of the dark place into which he was slowly sinking. He needed to convince the experts that his brain still had the ability to manoeuvre him and the Love Machine safely round the track at quite frightening speeds. It was a constant, frustrating battle.

'I went to Auckland and the specialist advised me about the long-term damage I could do. I felt they needed to do something comparative. I wasn't that good at school. I should have taken my school reports to show them. My cognitive skills were very good, which showed I was reacting well. I felt if they had put me on a bike that would have been the best way to test me. At the end of more tests they said I couldn't ride. I went back three times and I couldn't pass the test.'

Even when he did get the all-clear to resume racing after a year, his life remained empty and unrewarding. Mentally he wasn't in the right state to be racing. He'd joined the Kawasaki team and their experience of running road bikes was limited. Political problems with the team and his shattered family life made racing a chore. It wasn't like the good old days when he was the top ride for Suzuki and his father made sure everything he needed was procured and delivered. There was still a big hole in his heart and even racing couldn't fix it.

'Motorbikes were the only thing in my life. They gave me so many positives. I got a ride for Kawasaki New Zealand but I wasn't in a good frame of mind. My mechanic did some stupid things. In my first ride back my rev counter fell off and jammed between the forks and I crashed and ended up needing a knee reconstruction. I thought, fuck everything. I was back riding but it was just not working. I went away and turned into a party boy. But I was in turmoil inside.'

Just how that turmoil was going to be extinguished was a massive worry. Getting back on the bike had not been the panacea Love had hoped. Racing just wasn't doing it for him. He was still angry. He was still bitter and he was still confused. He couldn't find any way to channel the rage. The inspiration wasn't coming from within. So as luck would have it, it came externally.

'A couple of things clicked. Some people said some things and that gave me answers. I started hanging round some positive people. I copped some nasty stuff on the chin but once I processed it and learned about it, I realised it was true – I am responsible. Someone said to me that the only difference between a rut and a grave is the depth. That stuck with me. Another friend said to me, "Jared you are a naturally talented rider, but you are a whinger. You have had a disgraceful rough patch but get over it." It made me realise that I was responsible for all the stuff I had been doing.

'I got another opportunity. Dad bought me another bike and all of a sudden I was back racing for enjoyment and to be with my friends again. I forgot what a pig-headed, determined mongrel I had been when I was winning races. I went back to get my life together. I thought I was lazy and got stuck into it. I returned with the same bike the next year and started beating the factory boys. I was stoked. That led to me getting a ride for Honda.

'Losing the ride for Kawasaki, a lot of bad stuff went on. Everyone said I wasn't right after my accident but they didn't know how much shit was going on in my life. At the time it was heinous. I was an angry little man and I couldn't tell anyone. I got third in the nationals with the bike Dad bought me.'

And that was it. The power of a few home truths had rekindled the competitive fires. The dream of racing in Europe was a reality again. He had rediscovered his desire to be the best and make it to the big-money league. His success led to a contract with Honda and by 2004, Love was the name being whispered in the pit lanes.

Yet, he still felt he needed to put down a definitive marker to alert the racing world that he and the Love Machine were back living in matrimonial harmony. After everything he had endured on and off the track, there needed to be some closure signifying his emergence from the dark. Strangely, the Paeroa street race in February 2005 seemed the obvious place to climb back to the top of the racing world. What better way to get closure than to win the race that almost took his life? It would be the ultimate riposte. There could be no better proof of Love's courage and ability than to win at Paeroa.

It was one of the best fields ever assembled at Paeroa, with Love beating both superbike rider Andrew Stroud and four-time Robert Holden Memorial winner Tony Rees. 'I invited my mother back to Paeroa in 2005. One of the people who had helped me get through, his baby died at Paeroa at the track the first year I went back. They broke up and he left his wife, Shelly, with five kids. So, I persuaded Shelly, my friend, to come to Paeroa. I wouldn't let her give me any excuses. I dragged her there. Just before the race I put her little boy's name under my name on the bike and I told Shelly I was going to race for her. It is easy to look at someone else's life and get motivation off them.

'I won at Wanganui a few weeks earlier and got about 30 texts saying I was fat. One of my mechanics told me I had a triple chin. So I lost 15 kg. I went back to Paeroa, looked great, felt great and I won. I didn't realise it had taken me five years to get back to where I was when I was 23. But I'm proud of myself now. I wanted to do it and I achieved it. I wrote down in my diary that I was back. It was like a big switch being flicked. I was looking good and people were telling me I was looking good. I was an aggressive mongrel. I was there to do a job. It was a weight off my shoulders. I got to do something inspirational in front of people who meant everything to me.'

If there is justice in this world, Love will get the opportunity he lost at Paeroa in 2000. And if he does, the outcome seems certain – Love will conquer all.

After winning national junior Motocross titles, Jared Love switched to road racing in the late 1990s and had his first success when he won the New Zealand Formula 3 Road Race title in 1997. He also won the 1997 New Zealand Endurance Formula 3 championship, in his debut season, earning him a nomination for the prestigious Waikato Sportsperson of the Year award. He was a creditable third in the Superbike class in 1999–2000 – his first season at that level. In 2005 he won the Robert Holden Memorial race in the Battle of the Streets series at Paeroa. In 2006 he finished fifth in the New Zealand Superbike series.

16

MICHAEL UTTING

All White 1992-2003

The tears flowed and the relief was enormous when Michael Utting finally sat in front of a group of strangers and confessed to being an alcoholic. There was just so much emotion to get out. There was more than 10 years of pain that needed to be released. He'd been lying to himself for so long that he had nearly forgotten who he really was. He knew, though, that the time had come for the deceit to end. He couldn't stay in denial when only the day before he had been at Auckland Airport watching himself on TV. He was the lead item on the sports news. But it wasn't a story to make him proud. He had been booted out of the All Whites for breaking a team curfew.

He heard the news presenter tell the country that the international career of Michael Utting, arguably the greatest goal-keeper ever produced by New Zealand, was in tatters. He slumped into his chair, desperately hoping that by keeping his head down, no one would recognise him. And as he burned with the shame, there and then, in July 2002, Utting vowed never to drink again.

It was a promise he knew he wouldn't break but one that he understood others may find hard to believe. Booze had taken a grip of Utting for the better part of the last 10 years. He hadn't gone looking for it. Growing up in Wellington, there was rarely any drink in the house. No one in his family had much of a taste for it. He was usually the life and soul of any party while at school, but he didn't need to be full of lager to play the clown.

No, booze came looking for Utting. As a teenager, he earned a place in Wellington's Miramar Rangers in the National Soccer League. Crazy sessions on the turps were all part of the culture. No one thought too much about it. It was the norm, and ever keen to fit in, Utting did his duty. Post-match fluid replacement wasn't isotope-fuelled sports drinks. It was a crate of the local brew. After a game it was considered discourteous not to polish off a crate in the changing room before heading to the bar where the real session would begin. It was a way of life for young men with a bit of spare cash and a desire to play as hard as they worked.

As Utting remembers: 'I never had alcohol in the house. My mum and family never really drank. In my late teens I was just a normal Kiwi kid that would get on it at the weekend. I was a bit of a wild guy, a bit hyperactive, but never a big drinker. When I got into football it just came with the territory. On a Thursday after training it was a night out. There was no point going to a nightclub when you were stone cold sober. In those days we would finish a crate of beer in the changing room.

'We would fly up to Auckland for an away game on a Sunday. You would play, then fly back and quite often we would get on it at the Airport Lodge or stay in Auckland for the night. It was a way to socialise.'

To Utting that's all it was – a way to socialise. But by July 2002, when he watched himself lead the news, it had become so much more. He was a slave to alcohol. He was no longer in control and probably hadn't been since his late teens. There was no point in denying it any more. In terms of football, he had lost everything. He knew it wouldn't be long before he lost his tenuous grip on other parts of his life. There was no one to blame but himself. And he knew that only Michael Utting could save Michael Utting.

As he flew from Auckland to Wellington on that fateful day, he had time to ponder where it had all gone wrong. He had time to assess how it was that three years before, his name was being chanted by 80,000 fans in Mexico. The football-mad Mexicans had appreciated the heroics of

Utting's performance for the All Whites against the USA in the 1999 Confederations Cup. They took to chanting portero, portero, which is Spanish for goal-keeper. It led to him being named by the local papers in their dream-team of the first round. There was Utting, the boy from rugby's spiritual home, named alongside 10 Brazilians. That was why he played the beautiful game. Not even alcohol could provide the same high as playing football on the biggest stage. That is what he lived for and that is where he thrived.

'I remember we were lining up before the game against Brazil and everyone was in the toilets shitting themselves and our captain, Chris Zoricich, said, "Utts, how are you feeling?" And I said, "Don't worry about it mate, I'm going to be the best player out there today." I was thinking, "If you can't enjoy this, there is something wrong." All those crappy wet nights training, this is what they are for. It doesn't get any bigger than playing Brazil, the best team in the world. I said, "If you score a goal we will win." We ended up losing 2-0 but there was no disgrace at all. I had a great game.'

It's hard to fathom, then, why Utting was prepared to jeopardise his greatest love for the much cheaper and less enduring thrill of getting smashed. But that was just it, he didn't want to jeopardise his football career. His alcoholism, particularly as he remained in denial about its existence, was unwittingly taking him down a dangerous path from which he couldn't find any escape.

That grip was so powerful, he almost let the honour of playing Brazil drift past him in a drunken haze. After his man-of-the-match performance against the USA in 1999, he was dropped for the following game against Germany. 'We had a night out and I came home half an hour late. I got kicked out of the team. A few of the boys were later than I was. I came in through the front door, though. I didn't want to hide from anyone. It was a day off and I had gone out and got smashed, as you do. The next day I had to speak with the management. Ken Dugdale [All Whites coach] gave me an out where if I told him who else was out he would change the punishment. I did the crime so I did the time. I wasn't going to dob anyone in.

'There was all this media interest in why I had been dropped. Then we played Brazil on a Friday night. The other goal-keeper had an average match against Germany where we lost 2-0. We didn't know which one of us was going to play against Brazil until quite late.'

Utting got the nod but it had been agonising thinking that he might have blown his chance all for the sake of a cracking night out. The penny should have dropped after he was left out of the side for the Germany game. Something inside Utting's head should have been making a lot of noise to signal that change was needed. But it didn't happen, which is why, three years later Utting found himself buried at the back of the Safari Bar on Auckland's Ponsonby Road. He and a handful of All White team-mates were on a sanctioned night out watching the World Cup final. The All Whites were in camp preparing for the qualifiers for the 2003 Confederations Cup. They were to be back in the hotel by 2 am. Utting had every intention of playing by the rules. But fate intervened and gave him an option that would test his resolve.

'After the game we went to get a cab. It could only take four so two of us missed out. If we had got in the cab I would have gone back to the hotel and gone to bed. But I didn't. I followed my mate into another bar. We got back late, and chucked a few things off the balcony. That got reported to the management.'

If that had been his only indiscretion, maybe, just maybe, he would have been extended a reprieve. He might just have been warned to wind his neck in and set a more fitting example for a senior pro. But there were more skeletons in his cupboard that the management unearthed.

'Three days earlier we had played Dunfermline in Wellington. The night before I went to see the physiotherapist and told him I was so excited about playing in New Zealand in front of my home crowd. I asked if he had anything to calm me down. He pulled out a bottle of Cognac. So I drank the whole bottle with him. Then he pulled out a bottle of whisky. I drank that myself. This was the night before we played.

'Apparently I was wandering round the hotel eating plants. My roommate had to come and get me. That got reported back to the management after my second offence in Auckland. I remember being on the plane back to Auckland after the game against Dunfermline thinking, what sort of

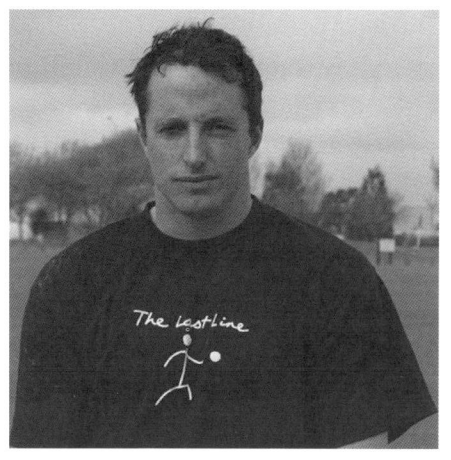

Michael Utting stares down the barrel of the camera after training. *Tony Whitehead*

sane person does this? And then realising I was obviously not sane. When you get away with it, you continue to do it.

'But when I got told I was being kicked out of the team I was so sad. I was very apologetic. I know now it was the best thing that could have ever happened. I remember going to the airport and waiting to get a flight to Wellington. The headline came up on TV – All Whites' goalkeeper gets kicked out. I was watching this and felt like everyone was looking at me. When you drink excessive amounts of alcohol, your self-confidence is low. I watched that and told myself I would never drink again. I said, "I'm never going to drink again then I am never going to let myself down." The next day I went to an AA meeting. I realised these people were in the same club as me. I said, "I'm Michael and I'm an alcoholic," and then cried my eyes out.'

After a decade of excess, Utting wanted to end his drinking with immediate effect. For many other alcoholics it's not that simple. The emotional tools are not in place to take on such a difficult project. The self-belief and willpower to facilitate change is often lacking. The slightest bump can knock the reformer off the wagon.

Utting, though, had once before tumbled down a black hole from which there appeared no recovery. So he knew the equipment to claw himself out was already in his locker. His confidence that he wouldn't break his vow stemmed from the fact he knew that admitting he was an alcoholic was not his nadir. That had come on 25 October 1995 when he awoke in a South African hospital with a broken neck. He was told he would probably never walk again and almost certainly would never play football.

It was catastrophic news for a professional sportsman. Yet, strangely, for Utting, it was almost a relief to be afforded an escape from the rut he had fallen into. In the years before he broke his neck, his life had not really been his. He was owned by the demon drink and he was punctuating the time between football games with sessions on the booze. It was a sad and empty existence but like all alcoholics, Utting was able to convince himself he was having the time of his life.

'I played a season in Australia for South Melbourne. At the end of the season they owed me money and they said, "If you sign another contract we'll pay what we owe you." I thought, "Stuff that, you owe me money and I don't want to be a slave to the game." So I went to South Africa to see my father. I had been to the UK but it was hard to get a work permit. I was a bit soft and in the UK you had to be tough. I was brought up without a male in my life. It was a hard upbringing.

'When I got to South Africa I ended up playing for Supersport United. I was drinking a lot of beer. I was a big binge drinker. I would go out and get shit-faced and convince myself that I loved it. I had a pretty lonely existence. I had a lot of friends when I was drinking. It was the way I was. I wasn't in a great state of mind. I was playing sport professionally and I was experiencing the highs and lows but never having a solid base off it.

'I didn't drink every day but when I drank I made sure I did it properly. I always ran out of booze. Once a month I would go in and buy a case of wine and it would be gone in three or four days. I bought huge glasses and I would drink it like lemonade. I would pass out and wake up on the sofa in my apartment with the cat sitting on me and three empty bottles next to me. And I thought, what a great night. I would ring up my mates in New Zealand and not remember it the next day. I would get these huge phone bills.'

It was a lifestyle that was always going to end in tears. They came when Utting was supposed to be looking after himself ahead of a big game that weekend.

'When I broke my neck it was a Thursday evening and I had just come home from training. I was going to have a quiet night because I had a game on the Saturday against the Kaiser Chiefs. It was going to be live on TV, a huge crowd up in Johannesburg and I was expected to do well. I liked the crowds and the passion the South Africans had for it.

'My mate was moving to Durban and he managed my local pub. About 10.30 pm he phoned me and said I had to come down. I was trying to get away from the drinking scene. But he came and picked me up and took me down to the pub. There were 10 shots lined up on the bar and I drank all of them. I was hammered. About two hours later we decided we would go back to my place and get some money – I had some cash – and go to the casino 40 km north of Pretoria.

'We got in the car and I think I fell asleep. I woke up in the hospital the next morning. It was a pretty frightening experience. My fifth and sixth vertebrae needed to be fused. I was told I would definitely never play sport again.

'It grounded me. Even though at the time I didn't appreciate what had happened, I look back now and appreciate it. You get your cheats out there who succeed and get to the top. There are bullshitters out there. Most of the time, if you do dodgy things it catches up with you. I thought I was invincible. I was a bit cocky and arrogant. That accident knocked me down a few places.

'My father arrived two days after the accident. He came into my room and looked at me and didn't think it was me. He thought he had the wrong room as my face was an absolute mess. It had swollen up like a balloon and I had a big crack down the side of my skull. When I came to a couple of days later and started to understand what was going on and was told I might not walk again, I wasn't fazed by it. I thought, "I'll get an insurance pay-out and do something else with my life. If I have to sit in a wheelchair maybe I'll go and tell people what a dick I am."

'I'd had enough of the life I was living. I'd had enough of playing sport and living like a dick. I had got to the stage where I thought I don't want to do this any more anyway. The car crash was maybe something that would force me to do something else rather than me choosing to do something else.'

As it turned out the crash did indeed force him to do something else, albeit temporarily. He was obviously in no condition to play football and the club's insurers refused to pay out as they said his accident occurred off the pitch. It left him with much to think about and while he was pondering his future he started to let himself go physically. Although he was gradually regaining his mobility and his strength, his normally chiselled physique was allowed to turn decidedly lumpy in the six months after his crash. He was able to walk, but the prospect of playing football was one he couldn't possibly entertain. Not just because of his neck, but also because he solved the interminable mystery as to who ate all the pies. His weight ballooned from 75 kg to 107 kg thanks to a diet of red meat that was washed down with copious quantities of lager. He was moored to the couch. His expanding girth was a sign of a sedentary life that was far removed from his pre-accident existence.

It wasn't a source of concern, though. There was no burning fuse ready to ignite a bomb of frustration at the prolonged absence of football. There was barely even a thought about football. Until, that is, Utting and his friends headed off for a night on the tiles about six months after his accident.

'We went to a rave one night. There were all these beautiful people there – gorgeous women – and I thought, I used to pull birds like that. And then I looked at all these beautiful guys and I thought, I used to have a body like that. My mate decided we had to get fit. For six months we trained our bollocks off. We didn't drink and we ate religiously well. Our money was going on the gym. My mate had a coin collect business and we would drive round collecting the coins and go to the gym together. I lost 34 kg in six months. I was super fit.

'Because of the mental state I was in after my accident, I wasn't really in shape to contemplate ever playing the game again. I needed to rest my body anyway and thinking that I was never going to play sport again, I think that helped me. I didn't have to worry about trying to get fit. I was living with my mate and his fiancée, and his brother and his wife. It was a house full of love and that is what I needed. It was pretty tough recovering from the accident, but I didn't rush it. I didn't have any expectations and that is why I think I got to the stage I got to.

'I was very disciplined. I would spend up to three hours a day in the gym and go to the park to do some sprints and kick the ball around.'

But he was all buffed up with nowhere to go, so to speak. Not just physically – mentally, too. The desire to play football had still not kicked in. His neck was feeling up to the challenge if required. It was the brain that was lacking the motivation. Despite having devoted most of his adult life to the sport, there was no intrinsic motivation shoving him back between the posts. Well, that's what he thought. It's just that the desire was lying dormant, waiting for a shift in Utting's tectonic plates to spark some activity.

That eruption came in Pretoria about a year after his accident. He'd gone to Loftus Versfeld to take in a game. And there, sitting in those vertigo-inducing stands, he effectively had an epiphany.

'I went to watch a national league game. It was Sundowns against Kaiser Chiefs. There were 45,000 people and I was sitting among them thinking, "I'm 27 years old and I am better than those guys out there. If I could play I would love to." There is nothing better than being out there. For 90 minutes you are a god. My biggest problem is that I underachieve unless I'm pushed or told I can't do it. That motivates me. If you get things easy, you can be complacent with it. But if you get told you can't do something, I'll prove that I can.'

And with the same certainty he vowed to stop drinking, Utting made the decision to return to football. The path back to the top flight was every bit as hard as the journey back to sobriety. There were more than a few hurdles to be cleared along the way. His neck was the biggest. Would it be able to cope with the rigours of professional sport? It felt good and he had medical clearance. But the medics can't ever guarantee. They can only offer odds.

Then there was the fact he was sans club. He wasn't quite persona non grata at Supersport United, but neither was there a whole load of trust in the bank. He'd broken his neck while indulging in a supersonic booze session only a couple of nights out from a massive game. Coaches, precious creatures that they are, can often suffer a serious sense of humour failure at such antics. His first step towards earning the trust of a professional team was to prove he was physically capable of performing at the top level again.

Utting eased his way back into the scene through a second division team one of his friends set him up with. His ultra lean frame was cruising through training. But then the game showed him how she could be a cruel and fickle mistress.

'I was training with a team in the second division. They were semi-professional. After a week I remember thinking I needed to give it up. I dived at someone's feet when we were one-on-one and he kicked me in the ribs. I ended up pissing blood for three days. I thought I could either lie down or I could see it as another tester. I believe you will get thrown curve balls and it is how you deal with them and adjust to them.

'I wasn't entirely sure how I could do a game. But then I thought, I'm glad nothing comes easy. It had taken me a year to get into that position. Not even kicking a football. I phoned my old club and asked if I could come and train with them. I wasn't being paid.

'I had actually been trying to sue them. They owed me money and because the insurance company didn't pay out, I was left with nothing. That was probably a good thing as it made me get off my arse and work.'

Good things had been in short supply for the last two years. Being allowed back to train with Supersport proved to be a luckier break than he could have possibly imagined. Fate, having been such a bitch, decided it was time to adorn Utting with a smile. Some say never give a sucker an even break. Utting bucked the trend.

'After I started training one of their goal-keepers got injured. And then another guy got suspended. I had looked really sharp in training but they wouldn't have given me a chance because of my history. I was out drinking when I should have been preparing for a big game. I was a loveable rogue sort of thing. But they were forced into giving me a game.

'It was a live game on TV against a team called Amazulu from Durban and that was my first game back. I felt as if I really had to do something. I felt as if my life was dependent on this. I took my chance and I ended up playing 17 games. We won the Grand Final and I got man of the match in that. We conceded a penalty in the 90th minute and that was the only goal I conceded in the cup.

'Former Manchester United and Liverpool goal-keepers Gary Bailey

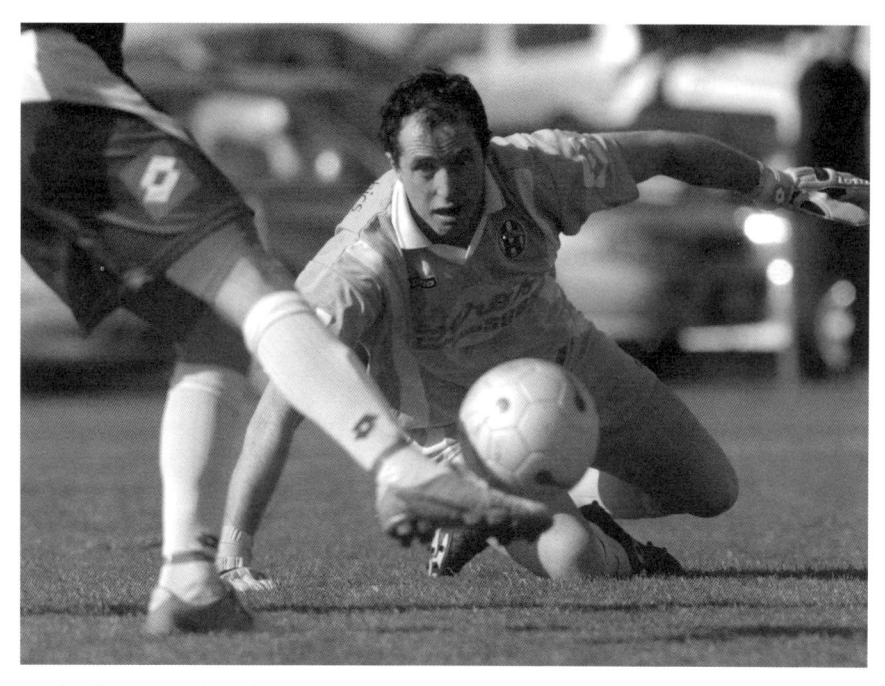

Michael Utting is kept busy during Waitakere FC's Northern Premier League match against Bay Olympic in September 2004. *Shane Wenzlick, Suburban Newspapers*

and Bruce Grobbelaar were friends of mine and they reckoned I could have played for any club in the world at that time. I was so fit and sharp. I conceded four or five goals in 17 games. Ken Dugdale, who was the All Whites coach in 1999, came to visit and he watched me. He was pretty impressed. New Zealand didn't have that great a standard of goal-keeping at the time. So I went to the Confederations Cup.

'Before the game against Brazil I had tears in my eyes. I had my hand on my heart as they played the national anthem and I remember thinking, "I'm playing against the best team in the world and I have achieved this after breaking my neck." It showed me that if you really focus and work hard you can achieve anything.'

That was a thought that came to the forefront of Utting's mind as he flew back to Wellington in July 2002. That he could do anything if he put his mind to it. Somehow, through the carnage, he could sense there was a brighter future waiting for him. His admission that he was an alcoholic gave him immediate clarity. It made him realise so much about himself.

It made him realise the only person he had been fooling during the last decade was himself.

'For a long time I didn't think alcohol controlled me. I thought I controlled it. I was always adamant I was in control. I could go out and have just one or two. I was an alcoholic for 10 years and it had to be something dramatic to make me stop. I thought I could control it. Now I realise I couldn't, otherwise I would have stopped drinking.

'If I hadn't been kicked out of the New Zealand soccer team I would have gone back to South Africa and ended up killing myself in a car crash. I used to drink and drive. Worse still, I would have ended up killing somebody else. It wasn't a good way to live. I had an agent in South Africa who owed me money and I had offers to go back and play. But I don't care how much money I could have made if it ended up that I was in jail being chased by some hardened criminal who liked the look of me. Money wasn't going to do much good then.'

Walking out of his AA meeting in Wellington, Utting had known darker times. The fact he was walking at all put him well ahead of where he was after his last spectacular fall from grace. But most importantly he had addressed the rot that had been at the core of both his slips. And now he wanted to make amends. He wanted to scream sorry and prove to all those he had let down that he was prepared to serve his penance. He knew he would never drink again and he knew he wanted to resume his football career. Being kicked out of the All Whites was not going to be his curtain call. He wanted another chance and he knew that to get one he would need to convince some sceptics that he had reformed.

'I knew I would never drink again. But I also knew that only time would show people. I spoke to Stuart Jacobs who was involved with the Kingz. I said I would like to play. They said no. But their goal-keeper signed for Blackpool. Ken Dugdale was coaching at the time and he said, "If you have admitted your problem and addressed it, I'll give you a go." I was totally committed.'

It had been a hard sell convincing Dugdale, though. His patience with Utting had worn a trifle thin over the years. The pressure was on at the

Kingz to get results. The perception, if not necessarily the reality, had to be of a club adhering to the highest professional standards. Any off-field nonsense would make the Kingz an even easier target. So it was a major call to give Utting a shot at redemption, and the fact it was made at all was largely down to Kingz assistant coach Stu Jacobs. For it was Jacobs who won the gaffer round.

'I met Michael in a cafe in Miramar shortly after he had been left out of the All Whites. We were struggling for a goal-keeper at that time so I mentioned Michael to Ken. Ken was humming and hawing because of Michael's past. Ken had been involved with the All Whites and had a few issues and run-ins with Michael. He took some convincing. It was a reasonably hard sell but we were able to convince him.

'We had to put a framework in place and create an environment that was right for Michael. We were aware we were taking him away from his support network in Wellington. We were taking him away from his AA meetings and people who were close to him.

'But a businessman called Dave Wilson who was involved with the Kingz had bought a property in Auckland and Michael lived there with me. That was part of the package we offered him – to stay out at Woodhills. We could keep an eye on him there. Michael has an addictive personality and that is probably what got him hooked on alcohol, but it also meant that when he got focused on something he gave it 100 per cent. He really trained hard and he really looked after himself.

'I guess as a player when you hear the name Michael Utting you immediately have respect because of what he has achieved in the game. He has probably been one of the best goal-keepers ever produced by New Zealand. But there were a few guys who were probably not so sure about what was going to happen off the field. I guess there was some concern about what would happen if the results didn't go our way or if Michael encountered some adversity. But he did a really good job. He did play that role of senior pro and we had no trouble at all from him.'

No trouble at all and a few months after he joined, Utting can remember some poignant words from Dugdale. 'Ken said after a game in Brisbane that I had played better than he had ever imagined. It was just me showing people what I could do. It was about me getting respect as a footballer and as a person.'

The key to Utting's redemption was honesty. Others would have taken refuge from their inner selves, too fearful to accept what they were. Utting has never been afraid to hold the mirror up and give the most frank account. Carrying only the truth he has been able to pick himself off the canvas again and again. Maybe if he had been burdened with some of the clutter that clouds the mind of bigger ego sports stars he would never have recovered from his accident in South Africa. He almost certainly would not have conquered his alcoholism.

'It is easier in life if you are honest with people. If you tell lies, you can look like a dick. I decided to confess I was an alcoholic. I was always scared what my team-mates thought about me. I was always trying to be everyone's friend. I worried they thought I was a dick and over the top. People respect me now because I don't drink. It is a nice place to be where people put responsibility on my shoulders. I would never have got that if I were still drinking. I achieved more when I stopped drinking. A lot of people in New Zealand know who I am and they look at my drink to see what I am having. I guess people would love to see me fail.'

Only the very small-minded would like to see Utting fail. The rest can see he's already done enough to be proudly proclaimed one of life's winners.

Michael Utting played for the All Whites 19 times between 1992 and 2003. His first taste of top-level football came when he broke into the Wellington-based Miramar United team as a 17-year-old. He was offered a contract with English club Crewe in the early 1990s but was not granted a work permit. Instead, he went to the South Melbourne club from 1993–1995 before heading to South Africa where he played for Supersport United. He signed to play for the Kingz in 2002, enjoying two seasons before deciding to step back and pursue other interests. He did, however, turn out for Waitakere United in the 2004–2005 Football Championship and then Young Heart Manawatu the following year.

17

SHANE HOWARTH

All Black 1993-1994
Wales 1998-2000

Thoroughbreds aside, Avondale Race Course wouldn't necessarily be the obvious venue to have a life-defining moment. It was for Shane Howarth. In July 1988, on Avondale Race Course field number six, he had to confront his deepest fears. Go face to face with the demons that had haunted him for the last 18 months.

It was there he had to make the bravest decision of his life. It was there he was faced with two paths. If he was brave enough to take the hard route his every dream could be fulfilled. If he wasn't, he reckons he would have been an angry, embittered, basket case to this very day.

It was torturous. But then again, since diving off rocks at Red Beach 18 months earlier, it was never going to be any other way. If only he had checked the depth of water when the tide was out, he wouldn't have been standing on a windswept field wearing his Marist colours wondering if the sport he loved could ever accommodate him.

It was a mistake any 18-year-old keen to impress the opposite sex could have made. Howarth had the sporting world at his feet in February 1987. He'd made all the Auckland age-grade sides while at Auckland Grammar and then St Peter's. He'd even enjoyed some time playing senior club football for Roskill. Then there was his other love, softball. He was more than handy at that, too.

Brimming with confidence and fuelled with the arrogance of youth, Howarth launched himself off some rocks on 18 February 1987.

'I thought I had done the sensible thing by testing the depth of the water. But being a youngster, and it being a cove, I didn't realise that I had tested the depth when the water had come in. So when I dived, it was at its lowest. I hit the bottom and I was travelling that quickly I split my head on the sand. I had pins and needles in my left arm. I got up and something was a bit strange because I couldn't drop my shoulders.

'They said it was a reflex action. If I had dropped my shoulders I would have passed out. I thought something was wrong. The old St John's boys tweaked my neck and said just jump in the Mini and get down to North Shore Hospital and have it sorted out. I stood up and blacked out. And my girlfriend said, "No way – get an ambulance." So they did.'

It was a decision that may sit as the best ever made on his behalf. If he had travelled from Whangaparaoa to Auckland in his girlfriend's Mini, it's unlikely he would be able to walk today. In the ambulance his neck was secured and he travelled in relative comfort. He was conscious and still unaware of how serious his injury was. That became clear when he got to North Shore Hospital and had his neck X-rayed.

'Half an hour after the X-ray they were packing my head. They told me I had broken my neck and not to move it. There are eight vertebrae in your neck and I had fractured the sixth and dislocated the seventh.

'I went into surgery that night and they fused the neck. I was three weeks on a traction bed. They had a halo on my neck and weights on it just to keep it still. What was fortunate for me was that at that stage New Zealand was leaps and bounds ahead in orthopaedic surgery.

'I was fortunate. I had to sign a form because the surgery was very close to my spinal cord. It was that or what else was I going to do? It was 10 hours of surgery. They said it went well. Once they fused it they said I would be able to walk around.

'I had played for New Zealand Under-17s so I was on the path if you like. I had played for all the Auckland sides all the way through. I had also played softball for New Zealand age-grade sides. I went to school to play sport really. It was devastating because the surgeons just said, "Look, we don't think you are going to be able to get back to playing rugby."

'They wanted to see how it set and how it fused. They kept trying to push me away from rugby. There had been an article in the paper about me and they knew how much it meant to me. Right at the end they said, "We recommend you don't play rugby again." They said, "We can't stop you but in our professional opinion we don't think you should." They said my neck was stronger than most but if I ever did it again I would be dead.'

It was a sobering thought. But not one Howarth could necessarily absorb and file away. Rugby meant everything to him. The thought of never playing again wasn't going to sit unchallenged. He couldn't just shrug and say, oh well. It was never that simple. His ambition didn't die when he heard his prognosis. He'd spent 18 years dreaming of being an All Black. It wasn't something that could be let go there and then. Every day after his accident he woke up to feel his heart sink as soon as he replayed the surgeon's words. There they were, loud and clear, reminding him that one moment of stupidity had cost him everything he wanted.

In the immediate aftermath it wasn't quite so hard to deal with the gaping hole in his life. He was still physically frail. The bones in his neck were still fragile. They needed to set and Howarth was required to wear an experimental collar that had been moulded around most of his upper body. Just like the surgeon's words, it was a pretty good way to remind him, every second, that he had broken his neck.

After three months he was allowed to ditch the collar. He went to work with his father making signs, and like most other Kiwi teenagers that winter, sat goggle-eyed at the inaugural Rugby World Cup. Maybe life wasn't so bad.

By August he was mobile enough and strong enough to play competitive softball. That afforded him an opportunity to at least quench some of his thirst to excel at the highest level of the sporting world. It was giving him social interaction, building his confidence and helping him realise that his accident hadn't robbed him of everything. But it could never be a surrogate for rugby. It could fulfil him only up to a point. Even if he made the Olympics playing softball, as was possible given his ability, there would still be an emptiness if rugby was to remain off-limits. When Howarth looked into the future, the only image conjured was of a sad man, angry at being denied his one big opportunity in life.

It made him hard work to be around. He was raging at his own stupidity. When he went to watch his mates play rugby it brought out the very worst in him. Eventually, his dad told him to get away from the game. He was told to go away and try to come to terms with his situation. Take on board the crossroads his life was at and try and make some positive decisions.

'Dad told me to get away from rugby. I was moody and sullen, thinking I might not play again. I was angry and bitter. All I wanted to do was play rugby and I wasn't allowed. I kept wondering whether I would ever play again. It was my life and then all of a sudden it was 50-50 whether I was ever going to play again. I was a pretty grumpy person to be around.

'It was my fault that I dived off those rocks. I tried to show off and do a great big dive. I couldn't blame anyone else but myself. Softball would never have been enough. I was telling myself it was enough. I had to keep telling myself to tone down the anger. I was angry at my own stupidity.'

But softball did have one massive benefit. It started to help Howarth realise that he was playing sport with no concern for his neck. He was able to fling himself around with little regard for his own safety. He was operating on instinct and there was no voice kicking in to advise against any potentially dangerous action. Diving head-first to make a base – no problem.

And that got Howarth thinking. If he could handle softball, then why not rugby? His body was responding just how he wanted it to and there was no interference from an over-protective brain. His neck wasn't featuring in his thoughts and it felt strong. It felt mobile. In fact, it felt about as good as it ever had.

But Howarth knew that comparing rugby with softball was a potential catastrophe. It was like thinking that just because you could handle a Toyota Corolla, you were ready for Formula One. His brain was ticking, though. His confidence was returning and the impossible had a slight feel of the possible about it.

'The massive bonus was softball because I could ease back into it. It was a good level and I had a good series that summer. I played for Auckland in the nationals. I was running, sliding head-first. That was defining for me because it got me thinking that maybe things weren't as bad as I was making them out to be.

'It was in the back of my mind that if I could play softball I could play rugby. I started going to watch rugby games and then I thought, "Hang on, how many people have broken their neck on a rugby field?" It's a one in a million chance I would do it again. But rugby is a whole lot different. I got through the softball season and my dad, who was a staunch Roskill man, said, "What are you going to do?"'

That was just it, Howarth didn't know. He desperately wanted to come back and play. But understandably he was scared. Very scared. The surgeon's words were always floating just a few inches below his conscious thoughts. They were easy to drag up whenever he started to get excited at the prospect.

No one was putting any pressure on him to return. If he wanted to come back and play it would be his call. It wasn't one that he was able to make until some sage advice from his physiotherapist gave him the clarity he needed.

'One of the physiotherapists said, "Either yes or no. Don't flounder. Don't go on the field thinking what if. Get on the field and play otherwise you are never going to know." It was a great bit of advice. It was totally my decision. My dad was staunch about rugby but said, "It's your decision – I will back you whatever you do. It has got to be 100 per cent your decision." Getting back into the sporting environment through softball helped me feel pretty good. So I asked if I could come back training.

'Dad rang up the senior coach at Marist, Kevin Boyle, and said that I wanted to come down and train. Kevin got hold of the Under-21 coach and told him I was going to come down and train but to keep me out of contact. So I went down to Marist and trained with them without taking contact. It was in the back of my mind that I had broken my neck. Then I started getting a bit more into it. I was dictating what I did. It was on my terms. Guys would run at me half pace and I was making tackles. I was testing different scenarios. It was always "Whenever you want".'

Shane Howarth

Whenever turned out to be July 1988 at Avondale Race Course No 6. His confidence had been built further by a few months of training with his Marist team-mates. He'd been bumped and bruised, but he'd never actually played a full game. He'd never flung himself into contact with the venom of old. This pat-a-cake, pat-a-cake stuff was all well and good. It added to his belief he could actually come back and play competitive rugby. But he needed to bite the bullet when he was called into the fray in Marist's game against Suburbs.

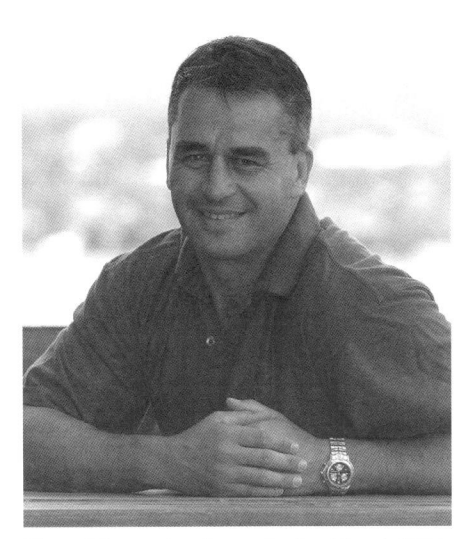

Shane Howarth at home in Auckland, 2004.
Fiona Goodall, Suburban Newspapers

'I was on the reserve bench. Then 10 minutes after half-time I said, "We might as well just do it now." I went in at first-five eighths. I was a disgrace for the first 10 minutes. I passed the ball as soon as I got it. I was a turnstile at 10. It was different to training. Those guys didn't know I had had a broken neck. All the Marist boys in training did. The Suburbs boys didn't care. It was a game of rugby and they wanted to win. I knew that and that is why for the first 10 minutes I didn't want to know. Guys would run at me and I would try and scrag instead of tackle them.

'After 10 minutes I thought this is ridiculous. I thought, "Either go for it and see what happens or turn around and walk off." It came to that kind of decision. I loved the game too much. I had to figure out what was going to happen. I took the ball off the next scrum and ran full tilt at them.'

The next five seconds were in slow motion for Howarth. It was almost Hollywood, life flash before your eyes, sort of stuff. Those five seconds took an eternity. 'I have never experienced anything like it. I have never had that experience of complete and utter fear of what happens when I get hit. It felt like about 10 hours for me. I got the ball off a scrum and I ran straight at this guy. I kept saying to myself, "I'm going to break my neck, I'm going

217

to break my neck." Not every rugby player is going to run in saying that. I was just trying to get over the psychological barrier of what happens.

'I got hit bloody hard. The whole ruck formed on top of me. It was panic. Complete fear. I got smashed and rucked and got the ball out. I stood back up and from then on it was full-on. That was the turning point. Now that I look back, and it is almost 20 years ago, I didn't need to have that. When you are 19 years old and have just broken your neck and you are getting back into a physical, contact sport you are thinking, this is make or break.

'When I got up I was thinking, "Why did I think that? You have already broken your neck, Shane. The chances of breaking it again are bloody remote." You have stupid thoughts.

'Even if I had gone in there and come out with an injury, I would have thought maybe this is not right for me. That was five seconds that defined what I was going to do with my life. It was a real feeling of fear but I was ecstatic. In the changing room afterwards I was climbing up the wall. I was jumping up and down. I had finally done it. I had realised that I could get back on.

'But it wasn't that games got any easier, because the next game I had exactly the same fear when I first ran on. My team-mates probably got pissed off because the first time I got the ball in every game I would just run. I wanted to test myself in different scenarios just to see. Probably the harder thing was getting back into the tackling mode. It is all right being tackled but it is a wee bit more important for me where my head goes.'

Confirmation that he had put his neck injury behind him came a month later, when he was called up to the senior team after just three games for the Under-21 side.

'My second run-on game for Marist was at fullback with John Kirwan on one wing, Terry Wright on the other and Bernie McCahill at centre. I was thinking, what have I done to deserve this? My senior debut was in late August 1988 against Eden at Liston Park. By then I wasn't thinking about my neck at all. It was gone because I didn't want to let myself down. It was funny the mental difference between running on and wondering if you are going to be all right to thinking that's John Kirwan on the right wing, that's Bernie McCahill at centre. Just don't fuck it up.'

Howarth would never forget those 18 months of pain, frustration and uncertainty. They were a source of motivation and at times a source of inspiration. Occasionally he would think about what he had done – recovered from a broken neck to play first-class football.

Really, though, his experience at Red Beach was something that he preferred not to give too much airtime. He knew he never wanted to be in that kind of mess again. He knew how much he wanted to play rugby. But he didn't spend hours dwelling on it. He came to a happy truce with his past, which was helped no end by the fact things were working out very nicely. As part of a successful Marist side he was noticed by the right people. In 1991 he was selected to play for Auckland. He was another step closer to fulfilling his dream of being an All Black. He was another step closer to burying the memory of Red Beach. Or at least finding the silver lining to that particularly gloomy and bothersome cloud.

Then, playing for Auckland in a Ranfurly Shield challenge against Nelson Bays in 1992, he was to get a horrid reminder of how lucky he was. For a fleeting moment, it was as if he was a Jedi Knight feeling a great disturbance in the force.

'I remember vividly we played Nelson Bays in a Ranfurly Shield challenge in Nelson and I tore my cruciate ligament. I came off the field and I'm not eerie, spooky or anything, but I thought something is not right. I was thinking something strange was going on. We were having a court session after and our captain, Gary Whetton, took me aside and said he had to talk to me outside. He told me my brother had broken his neck. I collapsed. I was in tears. Gary didn't know much. He just said I had to get on a plane and get back.'

When he got back to Auckland Howarth learned his younger brother, Arthur, had dislocated his fifth and sixth vertebrae. The two oldest Howarth boys had matching scars – both physical and mental. The whole incident had a profound effect on the elder brother. It brought back all those memories of Red Beach. And it also made him think that maybe someone was sending another hint. Maybe someone was saying that one of the Howarths had to go on to do something special. Prove there was a reason they both survived.

'My brother was an inspiration when he did his. His saviour was Zinzan Brooke. He was playing Under-21s at the top field at Marist. He went to make a tackle and the guy drove in on him. He put his head down on his chest and he heard a snap and he knew he didn't want to move. He knew what had happened to me. He knew straight away he had done his neck.

'Zinny came over and my brother said he had done something to his neck. So Zin said, "That's it. All of you get off the field and stay down there," and he stayed there with him. The ambulance came on while Zinny was out directing cars. It was phenomenal. The St John's guys wanted to move him and Zinny wouldn't let them. It was funny the difference. We have matching scars but he was in and out of hospital in a week. He had a far better collar and then he went back and played. He was my inspiration because I don't know if I would have gone back and played if I had broken my neck playing rugby. I broke my neck diving.

'As mentally strong as I like to think I am, my little brother was incredible. I made sure I went to watch his first game back. He tore straight into it again. So maybe it was a wake-up call for both of us. I thought someone was sending us a message that one of us has got to go and achieve something from here.'

It was obvious what Howarth needed to do. He had to become an All Black. There would be no better way for him and his brother to respond to their injuries. It wasn't talked about in the Howarth household. It was more an unspoken pact that they would both do what it took to achieve their goals. That pain and torment would have been for nothing, otherwise.

It also helped that Howarth's father was such a grounded individual who kept the family focused on what was important. Sure, his eldest son was doing great, but he could always do more. The importance of being humble was driven into Howarth. Which is probably why, when he was selected for the All Black tour of England and Scotland in 1993, there was only moderate celebration. It was right to enjoy the moment. Becoming an All Black is massive. When you make it six years after breaking your neck and after being told you should never play again, it can't really be quantified.

But it was celebration that was kept in check. It was not the right time to get carried away slapping himself on the back. He was still young. There would be plenty of opportunities to tell his war stories once his boots were in the cupboard. And besides, he went on tour but didn't play a test. That was his ultimate goal. To switch into self-congratulatory mode before he'd even won a test cap could have possibly derailed the whole mission.

Yet, even when the ultimate honour of an All Black test jersey slipped into his possession, there was still no acknowledgement within himself of how extraordinary the last six years had been. Howarth made his test debut in 1994 against South Africa at Carisbrook. He heard his name read out, but still the emotion was controlled as he was fearful that if he stopped to really think about how incredible his journey had been, it would have been hard for him to remain humble. So when he was selected to make his test debut, thoughts of his neck were buried. His immediate thoughts were the same as every debutante. He was worried about letting his family and friends down. He'd lived for this moment and once it arrived he instantly began to question whether he was ready for it. It was all perfectly normal. When he ran out to play the Boks in Dunedin, it never once crossed his mind that not so long ago playing for the All Blacks was an impossible dream.

But a few days later, when he came to watch the video of that game, it dawned on him just how special his achievement had been.

'I broke my neck in 1987 and it was 1994 when I played my first All Black test. The story had kind of moved on. The last thing I thought of when I got named was my neck. I had all the natural thoughts – I hope I don't let my family down and that kind of thing.

'Then in my first test it was either Grant Nesbitt or Keith Quinn who said when I took my first kick at goal – "Seven years ago he broke his neck. It's amazing he is here kicking a goal." Even some of the All Black boys said, did you break your neck? It was one of the South Island boys, I think it was Mike Brewer who asked. I showed him the scar and he said, shit, you did too didn't you? So when I watched the replay it hadn't really occurred to me that it was that big a deal. But when you sit down and

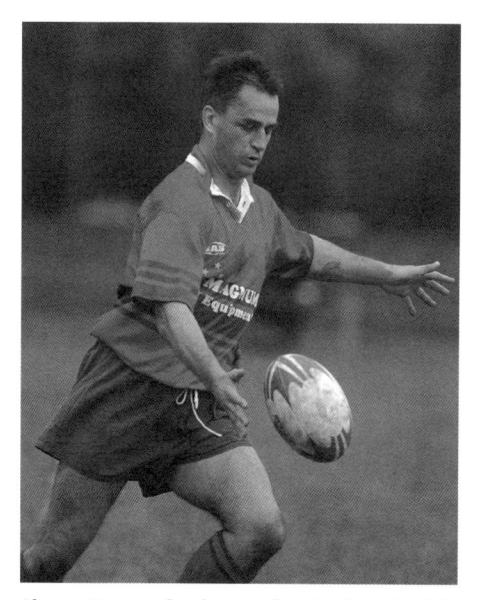

Shane Howarth playing for Auckland club Suburbs in 2004. He was player-coach there before landing the assistant coaching job at Auckland Rugby. *Fiona Goodall, Suburban Newspapers*

think about it, you realise it is not too bad coming back from a broken neck. To get back to that level of rugby, I realised how big it was.'

It was big. Huge, even. But there was no way Howarth was going to be allowed to bask in his glory. He kicked a conversion and five penalties in a 22-14 winning debut. A week later he knocked over another penalty at Athletic Park to clinch the series with a 13-9 victory and then at Eden Park he kicked all 18 of his side's points in the drawn third test. He got home after that test in Auckland having enjoyed the after-match glory that was lavished on All Blacks of that era. Everyone wanted to shake his hand that night. But before he could slip into a deep sleep, his dad breezed into his bedroom like the fiercest cloud and rained on his son's parade.

'After the third test at Eden Park I was living with Dad. I had kicked six penalties and it was an 18-all draw. But I had missed Brendan Venter one-on-one and he scored. I was getting all these plaudits. I got home a little the worse for wear and I heard the door creak. Dad came down and said, "You missed touch twice, you missed Venter and you missed another two tackles. That's not good enough." He shut the door and went back up to bed. If you have got level-headed people around you it helps.'

That need to remain humble, to keep striving for more, is what drove Howarth through a very successful football career. That and his buried memories of an 18-month stretch in the most inhospitable territory.

It made him stronger than most, which he needed to be towards the end of his career when he was caught up in what became known as

'Granny-gate'. Howarth was playing for the Welsh club Newport in the late 1990s and from there he was selected to play for Wales. In those days it was still possible to be capped by more than one country. He won 19 caps before a British newspaper revealed Howarth was not eligible to play for Wales. He understood he was, his eligibility coming through his grandmother. But the story caused a major scandal as at the same time another New Zealander, Brent Sinkinson, was also found to be ineligible for Wales while David Hilton, a winner of 41 Scottish caps, was found to have no heritage to link him with the famous blue jersey.

The scandal forced the International Rugby Board to tighten the eligibility laws and prevent anyone from representing more than one country. The British press enjoyed their usual feeding frenzy once the story had broken and Howarth was reluctantly thrust on to the back pages of almost every national newspaper. It was a torrid time, made worse by the fact New Zealand reporters were camping outside his grandmother's house in Auckland.

But just as it felt like it was getting too much, he could sit back and think about Red Beach 1987. Was it as bad as that?

'When all the stuff flared about the Welsh thing I thought, hang on, I have been through a lot worse than this. The crazy thing is England asked me to play for them against the All Blacks four months before I agreed to play for Wales. Why would I turn down the opportunity to play for England, a country I was totally eligible to play for and a country I would have earned far more money playing for, for a country that I wasn't? England were getting something like £10,000 a test in those days, which is a lot more than I got playing for Wales. That was the thing that annoyed me when all the shit happened. I was trying to get that across to people, but I never really got the chance. People just didn't understand that. I was really pleased that John Gallagher came out and said that he had only been in New Zealand for three months when they chucked him in the All Blacks. But when you break your neck and come back from it, I just thought, oh well. It grew me as a person.'

But nothing grew him in the same way as that day at Avondale Race Course in 1988. That was the day he shaped his own destiny by finding the answer to a question that had the potential to haunt him for the rest of his days.

'I had to get back and play rugby. Even if I had just gone out in the backyard and told my brothers to smash the shit out of me, I had to find out. If it came to that, I just had to see. Life would have been hopeless for me if I hadn't been able to get back on. I would be lying if I said I don't sit back every now and again and reflect on things and think about what happened to me in 1987.'

Red Beach could have crushed the spirit and sporting dreams of a talented young man. Instead it proved to be the making of an All Black.

Shane Howarth played four tests for the All Blacks and 10 games in total between 1993 and 1994, scoring a total of 135 points. He then had a brief stint playing rugby league for the Queensland Cowboys before heading to the UK where he played first for Sale, then Newport. While in the UK, he mistakenly believed he was qualified to play for Wales and earned 19 caps between 1998 and 2000. He then became the centre of a massive controversy when it was revealed he wasn't in fact eligible to play for Wales. He remains a much loved and respected figure in Wales, however, as he does in Auckland where he returned in 2004 to take up a post as assistant coach with the NPC team, who he helped coach to win the championship in 2005. His contract with Auckland has been extended through to the end of 2007.